ADVANCE PRAISE FOR
OFF OUR CHESTS

"*Off Our Chests* offers an unusually intimate and revealing glimpse into the reality of dealing with a cancer diagnosis—when you are in the unique position of playing every role: doctor, patient and spouse. At once deeply personal and bracingly universal, this book can offer cancer patients and healthcare workers alike the chance to meet one of life's most devastating situations with a rare sense of mastery and, yes, even hope."

KATIE COURIC
American TV Journalist

"This is a wonderful and engaging book - part memoir, and in equal part an 'autopsy' of the cancer establishment in this country. Written with immense care and kindness, it reminds us of how much we've achieved, and how much remains to be done."

DR. SIDDHARTHA MUKHERJEE
Pulitzer Prize winning author of *The Emperor of All Maladies*

"*Off Our Chests* is a must-read for anyone going through cancer. As with so many, I was blindsided by my cancer diagnosis. This book is a captivating and informative playbook for anyone thrown into the cancer game, but it is also a candid story about one couple's experiences with cancer which strongly resonated with me and my own recent cancer journey."

RON RIVERA
NFL Head Coach of Washington Football Team

"For those who face their own difficult diagnoses, this is a sort of *What to Expect When You're Expecting,* an invaluable guide for cancer patients and their families who may be struggling with what comes next. A powerful and deeply personal story of one couple's battle against breast cancer – a couple that happens to include a leading oncologist – told with honesty, candor and humor."

SUSAN PAGE
Washington Bureau Chief of *USA TODAY*

"This is an important book for the doctors and researchers in the pharmaceutical industry that illuminates the personal impact (both positive and negative) of cancer treatment. A remarkable book that anyone who has lived in the grim world of cancer will recognize, this is also the story of a couple's love and sacrifice as they bravely face an uncertain future together."

HON. PETER B. TEELEY
Author of *The Complete Cancer Survival Guide,*
U.S. Ambassador to Canada and Senior Vice President, Amgen

"Courageous, hopeful, heartbreaking, and a great read. I've known Dr. John Marshall, and Liza Marshall for more than a decade and *Off Our Chests* brings into light so many things that we all could learn from. As a parent, a patient, a doctor, a friend, or a caregiver, this is an incredible story from two of the best humans in this world."

MICHAEL SAPIENZA
CEO of Colorectal Cancer Alliance

"*Off Our Chests* is the kind of book I wish I had when I faced cancer. Written by the husband-and-wife Marshalls (he's an oncologist; she, the cancer patient), this book is perfectly balanced left-and right-brain, which is to say a highly useful guide to entering the territory of cancer land and an empathetic best friend to support you along the way. It's also a genuine love story—but not some sappy 'Love Story.' Recommended highly."

STEVEN PETROW
Contributing columnist at *The Washington Post*

"Every student, Resident, or Fellow who will care for patients with cancer should read this book! As a high grade, metastatic cancer 'survivor' (to date) I stepped between the pages of John and Liza Marshall's "*Off Our Chests*" and could not put it down. The open candor of dual perspectives from patient and long time spouse is captivating. Add the dedicated spouse's role as a senior oncology academic leader, and the tension is set. Each of us as patients with cancer enter roles as husbands, wives, and members of families suddenly facing our own mortality. The lessons from this wonderfully written 'gift' to each of us are invaluable."

DR. STEPHEN RAY MITCHELL
Dean Emeritus of Medical Education, Georgetown University

"The incredible journey of what happens when the accomplished spouse of an eminent oncologist develops an oft-fatal cancer. I laughed, I cried, I identified. Together they teach us the way forward."

DANIEL D. VON HOFF, M.D., F.A.C.P
Medical Oncologist, Translational Genomics Research Institute/City of Hope

"A must-read, inspirational memoir that will resonate with all those touched by cancer. Liza and John share personal reflections and insights into the cancer journey, and provide deeply meaningful perspectives from the patient, caregiver and oncologist point of view."

MARTHA RAYMOND, MA
Executive Director, GI Cancers Alliance and Founder, Raymond Foundation

"Off Our Chests" is 'Edutainment' at its best. This book provides a unique, valuable perspective that will be of great interest to oncology health care professionals and their patients."

NEIL LOVE, MD
President, Research to Practice

"In *Off Our Chests,* we are invited into the lives of Liza and John as Liza shares the cognitive dissonance of a young wife, mother and community activist with a serious triple-negative breast cancer, and husband John chronicles his dual roles of caregiver and world-renowned oncologist. The startling honesty, humor and intimacy of their writings are magnetically binge-worthy, as they open the kimono of Liza's threatened survival remodeling their marriage and careers, no holds barred."

DR. JOYCE O'SHAUGHNESSY
Chair, Breast Cancer Program, Baylor University Medical Center, Texas Oncology, US Oncology, Dallas TX

"This book is both a practical roadmap for cancer patients and caregivers and an inspirational story of a loving partnership between one of those patients and her caregiver, who just happens to be an oncologist. As such, it's a must-read for patients, but also medical professionals, advocates and everyone who has been touched by cancer."

CAROLYN ALDIGÉ
Founder and CEO, Prevent Cancer Foundation

"Dr. Marshall and Liza's account of their journey, from both the patient perspective, and just as importantly, the caregiver's perspective, is an honest, emotional, enlightening, and at times, page-turning glimpse of the ups and downs and the never-ending decision-making that follows a cancer diagnosis. It's heart-wrenching to hear from an oncologist-turned caregiver as he navigates his wife's journey with breast cancer and begins to appreciate what his own patients and their caregivers go through, and the enormous ripple effect that it has on so many people.

Anyone who has cared for a loved one with a cancer diagnosis will find their story brutally honest and hopeful at the same time."

JULIE FLESHMAN
President and CEO, Pancreatic Cancer Action Network (PANCAN)

"Liza and John Marshall have captured in vivid detail all that I felt and experienced after my stage 3 triple-negative breast cancer diagnosis in 2009. From the symbolism of the tattered pink ribbon on the cover to the post-traumatic stress that every caregiver and cancer patient eventually comes to know, their breezy style and wit captures the roller coaster that every cancer diagnosis brings. This book is an essential read."

JENNIFER GRIFFIN
National Security Correspondent - Fox News

off our

chests

To Ramon Parsons,
With great respect and admiration,

John Marshall

Liza Marshall

A CANDID TOUR THROUGH
THE WORLD OF CANCER

off our
chests

JOHN MARSHALL | LIZA MARSHALL

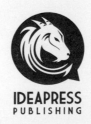

IDEAPRESS
PUBLISHING

IDEAPRESS
PUBLISHING

Published in the United States by Ideapress Publishing.

Ideapress Publishing | www.ideapresspublishing.com

Cover Design by Lindy Martin, Faceout Studios

Interior Design by Jessica Angerstein

Cataloging-in-Publication Data is on file with the Library of Congress.

ISBN: 978-1-64687-048-6

Disclaimer

Years alter one's memory but not one's feelings. While what we recount is how we remember things happening, we realize that our memories may not be completely accurate. We are sorry for those moments in *Off Our Chests* where our memory is imperfect.

SPECIAL SALES

Ideapress books are available at a special discount for bulk purchases for sales promotions or corporate training programs. Special editions, including personalized covers and custom forewords, are also available. For more details, e-mail info@ideapresspublishing.com or contact the author directly.

To Charlie and Emma

Contents

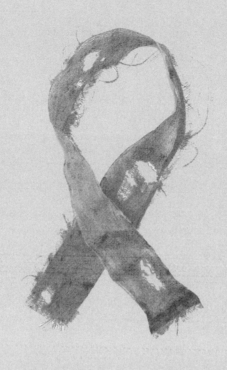

PART 1

Hail to the Queen

Breast cancer did not always irritate me. At first, it was simply one of the many cancers I had to learn about in my fellowship, essential knowledge required of all oncologists, especially because breast cancer was second only to lung cancer on the list of women's cancers. I was lucky that some of the true world leaders in the field were my teachers and mentors, and boy, did they make sure I knew my stuff. Maybe this is where my irritation started: They saw breast cancer as more important than others, requiring that we fellows attend all the breast conferences while considering that the other disease meetings were optional.

I was impressed by how smart all the breast doctors were; they had so many facts at hand, backed with a seemingly endless supply of data to support refined, effective therapies for virtually every conceivable clinical scenario. As fellows, we were expected to master those details and recite them in return. Failure to do so resulted in more than a ruler across the knuckles; public shaming was the favored form of punishment. They made sure we knew that they thought the other cancers, such as colon, pancreas, or lung, were for the less sophisticated student. The apparent reasoning was that there was not much to learn beyond a few basic treatments and palliative care for the inevitable end-of-life management.

As a lifelong sympathizer with the underdog, I became a GI cancer specialist, choosing to focus my career on the most common, most deadly, and most unsavory group of cancers on our planet. In my sure-of-myself, I-can-do-anything-if-I-set-my-mind-to-it way, I was determined to show those breast doctors that we could succeed, too, and that they were not smarter—just better funded. Sure, I realized that reaching my goal would require a major change in culture, from massive reallocation of research funding to broad changes in public perspective. As I watched the dominance of breast cancer strengthen—more Race for the Cure events, more pink ribbons, more high-profile celebrities signing on to help what I increasingly saw as "their" cause—the more determined I became.

I quickly came to see the ubiquitous pink ribbons as the enemy, a symbol of unfair focus in our field. Breast cancer comes first, and the rest of us get the leftovers. Would increases in research for GI cancers mean sacrifices in breast cancer funding? Maybe, but so what if it did? The breast juggernaut was miles ahead of the rest of us. It was our turn, and we needed a chance to catch up.

Lacking a strategy, ignoring the risks to my career, unable to suppress my feelings, I began slipping my anti-breast-cancer message into every dinner party, every lecture, every grand rounds,* every video, every interview. I preached my gospel of resentment and jealousy of breast cancer to anyone who would listen. It evolved into my brand, and, as validation, former audience members recited my "brown ribbon" jokes back to me. The angry glares from my breast colleagues, including some of my best friends, confirmed that my message was being heard. I was sure that if enough people in high places heard my message, I could put the breast cancer machine in its place.

Thinking back now, if I actually had succeeded, Liza certainly would be dead.

---

*Grand rounds are lectures typically delivered in academic medical centers by visiting speakers to educate medical trainees.

After I became relatively known in my own field of colon cancer, I often attacked the breast cancer establishment. Here's an excerpt from a sermon disguised as a lecture that I delivered many years ago....

"Updates in Colorectal Cancer"
Department of Medicine Grand Rounds
University of Somewhere
March 2004

I would like to begin by thanking the organizers for inviting me to give grand rounds for your department. It is a great honor to be here representing Georgetown University, and it's particularly heartwarming to see so many of you turn out for my lecture despite the rough weather today. I know how busy everyone is, and I hope that our time together can be meaningful, helping to ensure that you are up to date on the latest treatments for colorectal cancer. And for those of you in training, you med students, residents, and yes, even fellows, I hope that my words can either interest you in our field or, more likely, confirm why you wisely are going into dermatology.....

For starters, what is the most important cancer on our planet? Come on, you amazing test takers, anyone? Let me give you some clues. Which cancer type has by far the most funding? Which cancer are we racing to cure? Which one has an entire month dedicated to raising awareness?

Yes, of course, it's breast cancer—the queen of all cancers. Hail to the Queen! OK, what color is the breast cancer ribbon? Correct, pink! Clearly everyone knows that one. Every "Breast Cancer Awareness Month," formerly known as October, the entire National Football League turns pink; every flight attendant wears a pink tie or scarf; every cancer center lobby is decked out in pink for the annual breast cancer festival! OK, next question, what color is the colon cancer ribbon? Come on, you in front? Brown? God, I wish it were a brown ribbon—wouldn't that be great? Better still, it should be in the shape of a curled-up bowel movement, and how about this…wait for it…it should be scratch and sniff!

Obviously, I'm jealous of the success enjoyed by the breast cancer world, jealous of their funding and their pink ribbon brand on everything. They always have better drugs, better outcomes, and flashier advocacy. We GI cancer people are forgotten, the stepchildren living under the stairs—frankly, I am surprised you even turned out for this lecture. Why haven't our patients and advocacy groups risen up, pitchforks in hand, demanding more funding, better screening, better outcomes? Some say it is because no GI cancer patient survives to tell the story. Others say we GI people are too segmented and fail to speak with one voice. Maybe GI cancer patients sense the hopelessness associated with their cancer—advocacy efforts would only be wasted breath.

What evil, communist-loving, angry troll could possibly be against curing breast cancer? Even the Grinch, who notoriously stole Christmas, ran in the Whoville 5K to raise money for breast cancer. What loser would do otherwise?

You are looking at him.

Breast cancer has become almost sacred, untouchable, and yes, I am committing blasphemy right in the heart of the Bible Belt. As you can tell, I feel strongly that the time has come to rebalance our investments, not to take away from breast cancer research but to make equal the funding and support for all cancers.

Do you all know that over $100 million annually since 1992 is appropriated in the Department of Defense budget exclusively for breast cancer research? How on earth did our government decide to include breast cancer research in the same budget as bombs and tanks? This effort began *in the mid-1970s when First Lady Betty Ford came out about her breast cancer. She broke social norms of the time and persuaded Congress to insert big bucks into our Department of Defense budget specifically for breast cancer research, I suppose, by arguing this was in our national security interests. No one in Washington will ever have the nerve to cut breast cancer research funding out of the DOD budget. It would guarantee defeat at re-election. Cut the National Cancer Institute budget, sure, but never breast cancer funding.*

Why does this matter? Because, like moths to flames, researchers are drawn to grant money, and all their research has yielded impressive results. Over 90 percent of all women diagnosed with breast cancer will live five years or more. Most of them will be cured. Sure, the breast machine has real challenges. For example, they recently defined a sub-category called triple-negative breast cancer that rivals even the worst of the GI cancers, but triple-negative is not that common. Maybe our government could wake up and realize that most of the military is actually male and unlikely to get breast cancer. So maybe they should spend some of their seemingly endless budget on GI cancers before they invest even more to research triple-negative breast cancer.

Avon, African American Breast Cancer Alliance, Breastcancer.net, Breastcancer.org, Komen, Susan Love, National Breast Cancer Organization, National Breast Cancer Foundation, Men Against Breast Cancer, Mothers Supporting Daughters with Breast Cancer, probably even a group called Golden Retrievers Against Breast Cancer. Everyone is interested in beating breast cancer.

Why am I angry about the success of breast cancer research? Just yesterday I saw twenty-seven patients, each with a diagnosis of a GI cancer. The youngest was twenty-six, the oldest was eighty-seven, men and women, young and old. Of the twenty-seven, twenty will die on my watch, most within the next year. What is especially painful for me is that, aside from their family and friends, no one really notices. No one is organizing marches or fundraising for my patients. We are all too busy dusting off our pink ribbons for the next breast cancer event to notice the steady stream of people with other cancers dropping like flies.

Only recently have we embraced the fact that cancer is not one disease. The more we learn, the more we see just how unique each cancer is, meaning that lessons learned from one cancer type rarely apply to others. This basic principle took our multi-billion-dollar research industry years to actually comprehend and even more to embrace. (We are surprisingly slow.) As each cancer type becomes more complex, we physicians have had to respond by becoming even more specialized.

Most major cancer centers divide into teams, each with an interest, better yet a passion, for one particular kind of cancer. My new job as chief of our division is a lot like a baseball manager's, needing to field a team where players are very specialized—starting pitchers, relief pitchers, closers, catchers, infielders, outfielders—all working together but playing their individual role. Our team needs breast docs, lung docs, lymphoma docs, colon docs, etc., to provide the best care for our patients. As is true of baseball players, I have come to notice that people interested in one type of cancer have similar personality traits.

Breast cancer people never stop talking. Every point, even the smallest detail, requires a lengthy discussion of the pros and cons. Their clinics take forever—our group demands ninety minutes for a new patient visit when the rest of us can do it in sixty. What are they talking about? For God's sake, get on with it. Every breast study that was designed to produce a definitive answer instead produces more nuance that then requires more discussion. They pick every little bit of data apart and get drunk on data overload, but still act as if it was the last bit of new evidence they were ever going to see. Breast docs drive me crazy.

Lung cancer docs are hardened, tough, mostly men. It is a bad disease, and patients die quickly from this obviously self-induced cancer—except when it isn't. Lung doctors are non-judgmental, cool, unemotional.

Hematologists are the smartest members of our team. Just ask them! They have to be hardworking and fast on their feet because of the aggressiveness of the cancers they treat. Unlike many of us, their hard work has a good chance of fixing people. They are full of themselves, a bit like peacocks.

GI oncologists are the Gryffindors of the cancer world. We are by far the best humans God ever created: caring, loving, trying very hard, knowing we are going to fail ultimately, ever hopeful. We don't mind the smell of poop. Colon cancer is just plain gross—at least that is the public perspective. The fear of a diagnosis (the bowel prep alone freaks people out) and the fear of having an ostomy for life (actually pretty rare) are so great that many never get screened. Even my good friends who know very well what I do for a living regularly ask me, "Do I really have to be screened?"

"No," I calmly reply, handing them my business card, "but I can see you next Tuesday."

Of course they should get screened! Can you imagine a woman admitting that she had not had her mammogram? It never would happen.

Bear with me just a bit longer because I need to make one more point. Our center was originally a GI-focused center—we cared for Vince Lombardi. He had moved to D.C. to coach the team then known as the Redskins, and like all things (except Joe Gibbs) that touch the Wash-

ington Football Team, he died. Our early faculty were among the great GI cancer pioneers.

In 1988, all things changed. Marc Lippman joined our center as the director the same year I started as an intern. Marc is a world leader in breast cancer. He brought more breast researchers to Lombardi, following the ever-growing mountain of breast research dollars, and it was transformed into a globally recognized leader in the field. Pink ribbons were the norm. Fliers advertising "Look Good, Feel Better" programs just for breast patients were posted at every elevator. In the middle of the clinic waiting room that we all share, we built the Nina Hyde Room, funded by breast cancer philanthropy and dedicated to the Washington Post fashion editor who died of breast cancer. Technically, the space was meant for everyone but was intended specifically for breast cancer patients. There was no subtlety to it; breast cancer ruled!

Take a minute to reflect on this. Have you ever thought how a cancer patient who does not have breast cancer feels when he or she sees all the pink paraphernalia, all the resources dedicated to one cancer? They rarely express their resentment—too put down, too tired, too jealous. Second-class citizens. Not worthy. Non-breast-cancer patients do not say anything. I feel strongly that we should help them find their voice.

So the next time you see an ad for breast cancer research, an offer to participate in a three-day race to cure, or read yet another New England Journal article proclaiming yet another therapy that further improves the outcomes of breast cancer patients, you might reflect on the rest of us. We are literally dying over here. Without advocacy, without dedicated research funding, we will never move the bar for our patients. I ask you here today to join our choir, be the voice for the non-breast-cancer community, help break the spell, hear the cries of those continuing to *suffer, not previously heard above the hosannas for breast cancer. We too need funding for research. We too need to look good, feel better.*

I know a few who have heard my rants and joined the crusade. One person made me a ceramic brown ribbon, probably in a beginner's pottery class. It is nearly a foot across. It is clearly brown, it is clearly a ribbon, and it resembles a bowel movement—a good one, not a mushy one. It greets all who enter my office.

If only it could have been scratch and sniff.

OK, then. Before I use all my hour ranting about breast cancer, maybe I should actually share our research on colorectal cancer....

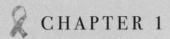 CHAPTER 1

The Announcement

T hanksgiving week of 2006 came with its usual flurry of school and family activity. The regular routine involving Thanksgiving pies pickup on Monday, Grandparents and Special Friends Day on Tuesday, and then no school on Wednesday, every mother's dream as she schedules the shopping, cooking, and other preparations for the big event on Thursday. We usually went to Kentucky for Thanksgiving to see John's family, but this year we changed our plans and stayed home. We invited my parents and sister, Lucy, as well as Dr. Claudine Isaacs and her family for Thanksgiving dinner. Claudine is a breast oncologist at Georgetown Hospital and a friend of ours since she and John did their oncology fellowship together at Georgetown in the early 1990s. It was going to be a hectic week as we prepared to feed eleven people what we hoped would be a gourmet feast.

When I woke up Monday morning, my major focus was on logistics and figuring out the answer to the question: How was I going to get it all done? I got the kids to school and came home to try to clean things up before heading back to supervise the Thanksgiving pie distribution, a school fundraiser I had organized that year.

John called mid-morning to go over the logistics for the evening, getting one child to basketball practice and another to a piano lesson, fixing dinner, feeding the dog, purchasing the groceries for Thursday's meal. As we chatted, he became distracted by a colleague entering his office. "Dr. Liu is coming into my office. What can I do for you, Dr. Liu?" he said cheerfully. I glanced at my computer, quickly scanning incoming e-mails while his attention was elsewhere, assuming he and Dr. Liu had some business to transact.

"You have breast cancer," I heard my husband the oncologist say. His voice was incredulous, choked. I jolted back to attention. "You're kidding," I said. Not a very funny joke, but John likes to push the envelope and say shocking things to people to get a laugh. Sometimes they fall flat; this one was falling flat. Then I heard him talking to Dr. Liu in the background and asking what she was showing him. "No, I'm not," he continued. "Minetta just handed me the pathology report from that breast tissue specimen research you did, and it shows cancer cells in your lymph system." I really couldn't process this. Dr. Liu wasn't my doctor. She was a colleague of John's, a breast oncologist at Lombardi Cancer Center. I knew her socially from work events, but I had no idea why she would be appearing in John's office in the middle of a workday to tell him I had breast cancer.

* * *

A brief history of my breasts. There were two of them, and they had been relatively trouble-free over the years—although I was the last girl I knew to acquire them. They had always been small, a point of some disappointment for me, which probably turned out to be a good thing later on. My mother, who did not have the problem of small breasts, tried to make me feel better by telling me that breasts were mostly fat, and because I was thin, mine were not large. That was small comfort when I was a teenager and large or at least average-sized breasts seemed to be what interested most teenage boys. Eventually, when I went to college, I met men who seemed to be able to see beyond (maybe above?) the breasts. I think John was actually attracted by my general body type, not that he would have complained. I have known women whose husbands asked them to enlarge their breasts, but it would be out of the question for John to ask me to alter my body for his pleasure. To be honest, he probably would be afraid to ask because he knows that I am strongly opposed to unnecessary surgery and that I have strong feelings, not positive, about a society dominated by the opinions and preferences of men. And he knows that I can be pretty fiery when pushed.

So we have made do over the years with what the good Lord gave me and enjoyed a mutually gratifying sex life. The physical health of my breasts had been relatively good. I had a cyst in my left breast in my early twenties, which occasionally became painful. My gynecologist recommended that I reduce my caffeine intake and take vitamin E. When I was nursing my children, my breasts served all of us well, and they both thrived. I had the usual issues of sore nipples, and my son did reject my right breast frequently, which the new mother bible of the time, *What to Expect When You Are Expecting*, warned might mean I had cancer in that breast. But after a few tears and a small bout of fear, I determined I was being silly, and we moved on. I wonder if he knew something then that I didn't.

A much more personal introduction to breast cancer came out of the blue—as cancer almost always does—in the fall of 2001. A friend of mine and the intrepid room mother for my son's third-grade class, Holly Richardson, pulled a few of us aside one day in the hall at school to say that she had had a mammogram that indicated that she had a mass in her breast and that she was going to have surgery. I was the only one in the group who had not had breast cancer, so I obliviously tempted fate and joked that I felt left out of the club. They all looked at me as if I was a dolt, which I clearly was, and one of the mothers said with a horrified tone, "You don't want to be in this club!"

Holly had her surgery a few days later, and when I next saw her, she told me that the surgeon had burst into tears when she gave Holly her pathology results: All of the lymph nodes they had removed were positive. I knew that meant it was bad, that the cancer had likely spread beyond the breast. I also knew that many people die of breast cancer, even those who are forty-six years old, and that surgeons don't usually burst into tears when giving patients their pathology results. (I made a note not to go to that surgeon in the future.) Holly was clearly panicked, and I told her that she should call John and get in to see someone at Lombardi, one of the best places to go in the United States if you have breast cancer. John greased the wheels for her, as he has for so many, and she was quickly seen and started chemotherapy. Things went well for about nine months, not counting the side effects of chemotherapy and radiation.

With Holly, a proper South Carolinian and pillar of every community she was in, you wouldn't know there was ever anything wrong. There were occasional glimpses into her fear that she would show a very few people. Once she asked John if this would be her last Christmas with her kids. (He assured her it wouldn't.) She kept up her full-time job as an assistant to a United States senator, and she acted as the primary caregiver for her two children, who were in third and seventh grades. She continued as room mother while also serving as president of the school Parent Teacher League. Holly's fresh baked goods appeared for almost every occasion in which she or her children were even tangentially involved. I imagine she continued to entertain and probably made food for people in need. Cancer still didn't look that bad....

That is, until the following summer when Holly's husband, Phil, called us from their car as they were driving to a picnic at a friend's house, taking whatever delicious food Holly had whipped up for the occasion. "Can I talk to John?" I handed the phone over. Phil told him that Holly's face had suddenly drooped on one side and that she had endured an intractable headache for a few days. John told them to go to the emergency room immediately. It seemed obvious that Holly had metastases in her brain, quickly confirmed by an MRI. She was admitted to the hospital so they could start more aggressive and directed treatment. John and I went by to visit her the next day, and she and Phil were clearly terrified. Who wouldn't be?

The next few months were awful for everyone. We all tried to help Holly and the family with food, a schedule of friends to keep her company at the hospital, whatever we could think of. Holly's parents sat in her hospital room looking both dazed and angry. Phil looked bewildered. Holly soldiered on, taking whatever treatment was offered, not letting on to anyone, even the medical staff, that she had gone blind, suffering a device implanted in her scalp to deliver the chemotherapy directly to her brain, trying to walk to the bathroom and avoid using the bedside commode because that was a concession to the cancer and undignified behavior. It was a portrait of desperation and courage and immeasurable grief. I did what I could, visiting Holly frequently, trying to help with her room mother role at school. John and I talked about her situation almost constantly. It was terrible to watch someone descend so rapidly, knowing there was little hope. Finally, on September 30, 2002, Holly died. Her standing-room-only funeral remains one of the saddest I ever attended.

While my own breasts seemed fine, the experience we had with Holly's short battle made the specter of breast cancer much more immediate and its potential deadliness a new reality. All her friends were left both numb and terrified by what we had witnessed, and we continued a sort of support group for several years not only to honor Holly's memory but also to lean on each other after the trauma. Her story still comes up frequently in conversations; her friends remind each other of details of how we found out what she had, how bad it was, how quickly she died, what things she said. We remember her incredulity that anyone would suggest she couldn't still be the room mother, even though she was clearly weeks from death. We continued to speak of her and our experience in hushed tones and looked at each other aghast as we relived it all.

In the spring of 2006, four years after Holly died, I was doing my monthly breast self-exam and found a hard lump in the upper-left quadrant of my left breast. I moved my hand away and then returned to the spot, palpating it again to see if I had imagined the hardness. I hadn't. My adrenaline kicked in as the panic rose. I reminded myself that I had had cysts before and this was most likely another one, but I knew there was a chance it wasn't, a chance that breast cancer had made its way to me. I knew I had to get it examined by someone with "breast lump" experience. First, I told John and asked what he thought I should do, not because I didn't know but rather because I wanted a judgment on whether I was over-reacting. "I'd get it checked," he said in a blasé way. We decided I should go first to see my gynecologist and have her take a look. After probing and asking a few questions, she advised me to see a breast oncology surgeon to have a further look, but she reassured me that it was unlikely to be anything scary. However, it's nearly impossible not to be scared and start the "what ifs" when you are sent to the next level of medical investigation.

I was remarkably fortunate that one of John's colleagues was Dr. Shawna Willey, a surgeon at Georgetown University who was recognized nationally and internationally for her expertise in breast cancer. She was sought out by many women in the Washington, D.C., area and beyond for her medical abilities as well as for her kindness, caring, and gentle humor—qualities often in short supply among surgeons. I went to see her almost immediately. She examined me and said she didn't think that the lump was anything scary, but she wanted me to have an ultrasound and a mammogram. The radiology report found that I had "an ovoid solid lesion measuring approximately 1.3 cm" and recommended a biopsy.

Dr. Willey sent me for an ultrasound-guided core needle biopsy the following Monday. The radiologist who performed the test warned me that the noise would be somewhat unpleasant and that although they would numb my breast, I would feel the pressure of the needle shooting in. It was a bit off-putting, having a piston-type device forcefully injecting itself into my breast several times. The radiologist was calm and matter-of-fact, but she knew that almost every woman who walks into her procedure room is afraid of both the test and what it will find, so she was also warm and soothing. A few days later, the pathology report came back, and Dr. Willey called to tell me. Diagnosis: "Benign breast tissue consistent with fibroadenoma."

Phew! Now I could go back to my regular problems!

Hence in late October that year, when I was standing naked in front of the mirror in my bathroom one morning brushing my teeth after my shower, I wasn't too panicked when I noticed that one of my breasts was swollen. I wasn't even sure it was. It didn't hurt or feel any different to the touch. I try not to be a hypochondriac, and I had never heard of breast cancer presenting with a swollen breast, so I took a second look and then asked John, "Do you think my right breast looks swollen?" Again, he seemed pretty nonchalant and said, "Yeah, maybe. You could have Shawna look at it." I called to make an appointment. When we met at Georgetown a few days later, she too seemed nonchalant. We chatted about our children and life, and she ordered a mammogram and an ultrasound. I headed down the hall in my hospital gown for the procedures, then raced home to attend an afternoon of kids' soccer games.

The radiologist's report on the ultrasound from that day concluded: "It is uncertain if this is a real lesion. The patient could return after the onset of her next menses, with the idea of performing a repeat ultrasound. If this lesion persists at that time, it should be amenable to an attempted ultrasound-guided core biopsy." Interestingly, the mammogram report stated that there was nothing suspicious. Mammogram reports have always noted that I have dense breasts and that it is harder to see changes in dense breasts. My mammogram report also noted that approximately 10 percent of all cancers will not be detected by mammography, my first encounter with percentages I did not like. Dr. Willey told me that she would like me to have a core needle biopsy, and we scheduled that for a few weeks later.

On November 16, 2006, a week before Thanksgiving, I arrived at Georgetown for my biopsy. I sat in the breast procedure waiting room, shivering and scared. I was now at the next level of medical investigation, which I knew could still turn out to be nothing, but it was getting harder not to play the "what ifs" game with myself and to keep a brave face.

Eventually John appeared, looking worried as he prepared to join me for the procedure. A few minutes later, a med tech called us back to a procedure room and helped me onto a table. She noticed that I was cold and brought me a warm blanket, which provided some comfort. Then nurses arrived with paperwork, one to affirm informed consent about the procedure, the second to ask about my interest in participating in a research study by permitting my breast sample tissues to be bio-banked for research. I didn't have to think long. I am married to an oncologist who has long advocated participation in clinical research. My belief system is grounded in the notion that people working together and giving of themselves will improve life for everyone. Plus, I love completing paperwork. (Yes, you read that correctly.) There is something so satisfying about knowing all the answers to the questions, so that was an easy yes.

The radiologist Dr. M arrived. She was petite and dark-haired with a gentle manner. Despite being a procedure room filled with metal instruments, the space was almost soothing. The lights were low so that the radiologist could see the screen, and the screen itself gave off a warm ambient light. I lay there as still as possible with the ultrasound wand pressed against one side of my right breast, while the spring-loaded needle once again shot in and out of the other side of my breast. The radiologist acknowledged that while she was using the ultrasound machine, she couldn't see anything in the breast, so she was following Dr. Willey's direction as to the target area. This complicated matters for the doctors and, of course, for me. After several passes at the breast with the spring-loaded needle, Dr. M wrapped up the process and reminded me that I should ice my breast for the rest of the day to keep the trauma to a minimum, an admonition I failed to follow, so I ended up with a black-and-blue breast for another week.

Soon that was going to be the least of my problems.

I don't know when I would have heard that I had breast cancer if I had been just another patient going through the regular channels. Because I agreed to have my tumor bio-banked and because my husband worked down the hall from the researcher running that study, four days after my core needle biopsy, I found out I had breast cancer from my husband. He knew it even before the doctor who ordered the test did. Dr. Minetta Liu had received the pathologist's report that there were tumor cells in the sample I had provided as a routine part of her study. (John remembers the details differently. In his memory, he learned of my cancer because he was accidentally copied on the pathologist's report.)

My guess is that with other patients, that information would have gone to their surgical oncologist, who would have called the patient with the life-changing information as part of his or her normal process. Dr. Liu would have gotten it, too, but I imagine she would have let the process go forward through the surgical oncologist's office, perhaps just checking to be sure the oncologist saw it and would follow up with the patient. However, as soon as that report appeared on Dr. Liu's desk, she walked to John's office with it when I just happened to be on the telephone with him.

Did other people married to doctors find out about their medical problems this way? Would this foreshadow how other chapters in my medical odyssey would unfold with John knowing things about my medical condition that I didn't? It wouldn't be all bad, of course, to have someone who knew about cancer checking in every day, watching over me and my care. But I didn't know if I felt comfortable with him being in charge of this either, even if by default. He's not inclined to keep his opinions on how we all should do things to himself. I had managed medical care for myself and the children pretty well thus far, and I didn't want to feel the need to check in with John or have the thought that he had all the information and I didn't. But maybe I would want to be told what to do. Did I want to know everything, or didn't I?

"Well, what do I do?" I said, my voice teetering a bit out of control. "You need to get an MRI and CT scan right away, this afternoon," John said.

"But I can't!" I protested. "I'm running the holiday pie distribution at school, and the pies are due there in two hours." I fretted about the pie delivery, the other mothers who had signed up, the chaos that surely would ensue without my organizational skills. "I have to be there."

John kept calm but was insistent. "I'll come and help, but you need to come in today."

I don't know if this is the approach he has with his own patients (not that he would step in and assume whatever quotidian responsibility stood between the patient and a necessary test). Nor do I know that other oncologists tell their patients a scan must be done the day the pathology report comes back. But here the intersection of oncologist and husband led to barely controlled panic and a call for immediate action. He might already have been trying to figure out how he was going to raise the kids alone. I had been complaining about neck pain for a couple of weeks, so he was certain the cancer had already metastasized to my cervical spine. Plus, Thanksgiving was coming in three days, and that meant waiting at least a week for anything to happen if I didn't go in that day.

I heard the panic in his voice and the unprecedented offer of taking time away from work to participate in a mundane school activity, so I accepted. I somehow got myself to the school in time to receive the pies and not to let on to those who were helping that anything out of the ordinary was happening, even as my insides roiled with shock. John arrived, and we organized and sorted the pies as quickly and calmly as possible, then exited.

John's appearance at school did not go unnoticed; our daughter, Emma, who was in fifth grade, ran across him in the front hall and was immediately aware that something was not normal. "What are you doing here?" she said. "Just helping Mom with the pies." John casually replied.

"Oh," she said skeptically, and she headed back to class.

John had called my parents earlier and asked them to pick the kids up from school. He told them what was going on. I wasn't up to talking to anyone or even saying out loud that I had breast cancer. I was spiraling, trying to keep everyone else's life normal while trying to process what was happening to me. And it did feel as if it was happening to me: *Here's what you have; here's what you need to do; here's where you need to go.*

And, always, *here's what happened to Holly.*

CHAPTER 2

The Calling to Cancer

I was born into a world where I believed the parental line that I could be whatever I wanted to be—equipped with basic innate gifts, amazing mentorship, love, support, and seemingly unlimited funds—not to mention being a white male. My mother's cancer was my first experience with disruption, my first real loss, a wound I carry that has never really healed. Our family's financial collapse followed a few years later. Between the ages of thirteen and sixteen, I had a crash course in loss. I learned what it felt like to have nearly everything one minute and to have lost almost all of it the next. I learned that our existence is fragile and requires constant vigilance to maintain, with someone always on patrol to guard against the wolves and to keep the mouths fed. The feeling of loss terrified me. I hate being cold, and I hate being hungry. I would never survive on the street or in the wild. (My family refers to me as the "Prince and the Pea.")

I became obsessed, and still *am*, with preserving and protecting our family and our way of life. I know sudden, dramatic loss can happen to anyone, no matter how prepared. My blood pressure rises, and my heart races at even the thought, pushing me to build even more layers of protection and put yet another safety net under us. Cancer taking my mother, quickly followed by our version of "Black Tuesday," was by far my most fundamental motivator in life. I was not going to let cancer hurt my family again. I was going to cure cancer, and I was going to provide financial stability for my family while doing it.

I was born in Frankfort, Kentucky, in 1961, between an older brother and a younger sister, and raised in Lexington by loving parents who made our house the magnet for the neighborhood kids. I attended the best school in town and took advantage of every opportunity available, from YMCA Indian Guides (certainly no longer a politically correct moniker) to basketball, soccer, and Little League baseball, as well as world travel. Always the showman, I organized summer backyard fairs complete with miniature golf courses and Halloween haunted houses in our basement. I kept the crowd laughing with a raunchy sense of humor typical for a ten-year-old boy with a smart mouth. I always knew I wanted to be a doctor because I loved science and seeing people naked.

My father was and still is the "fun" parent: creative, witty, warm, adventurous, and accepting of all shortcomings. Although he worked hard, he always left work at five o'clock to play with us kids. He loved boats and new gadgets. My father was not just an idea guy; he was a "big idea" guy—in my eyes, his most admirable trait. In one of his incarnations, he successfully developed farmland that was situated between small Kentucky towns and exits off Interstates 75 and 64, building themed strip malls with a Kroger grocery, a drugstore, and local specialty shops, bringing jobs and access to small-town America.

Even though I knew her for nearly fourteen years, and I was apparently a "mother's boy," memories of my mom are hazy, with vast chunks missing, maybe suppressed. What memories endure are almost certainly idealized; dead mothers become saints. My mother was in charge. She was the detail person for our family. She organized us and everyone around us. She made our home safe, warm, and predictable. She was the rudder in my father's boats—in fact, even though she never really liked the boats, they were named for her, each christened "The Lady Jane."

Mom set the standards we lived by. She was all about duty: to others, to God, to fulfill one's potential. She was respected, valued, and loved by all. Her love and care for others were at odds with a streak of narcissism. She was quite pretty, maybe more elegant than pretty. She loved fine clothes, traveling to Europe, and shopping in New York, eager to parade the latest fashions before our central Kentucky neighbors. It was important that we display our sophistication to show the rest of Lexington what the outside world was up to.

When I did well in school or other aspects of life, Dad was never over the top with praise, as so many parents are today. There were no trophies for participation in our house. His line was always, "If a boy like you does not do well, then who will?" Dad always bragged about me and my siblings to his friends, but praise was rarely directed to us. As a result, I developed my own set of expectations. I felt driven to succeed. With each new achievement in school, with each advance in my career, I got the same line:

"If a boy like you doesn't succeed, who will?"

As with so many sons and fathers, no matter what I did, I never got that longed-for trophy. I could only disappoint; I became determined to never disappoint—anyone.

Church was a big part of our life. As Baptists, we attended church Sunday morning, Sunday night, and Wednesday night. I sang in the Youth Choir, belting out hymns and anthems with my best church friend, Tim. We were so awesome that I believed a career in Broadway musicals was there for the asking. (I had not yet learned *never* to believe my own press.) At Calvary Baptist Church, I discovered that I love an audience.

The Baptist church tortures its young people by having Bible drills, an incredibly stressful public competition among teenagers. It rewards those who could find Bible verses the fastest, those who could memorize the most verses (no prize for understanding their meaning) and obscure Bible facts, hastily crammed just when your real schoolwork is starting to get hard. I hated Bible drills, but they turned out to be among my first public speaking experiences. To avoid the embarrassment of being unprepared in front of God and everyone, I did my best to know my verses, but when I didn't, I adopted the rescue technique to make 'em laugh. While Baptists did not allow dancing, it turned out they did like laughing.

I am forever grateful that Mom showed me where to find God, how to talk to God, and more important, how to listen for God. She lived her life following the Golden Rule: We tried to do unto others as we wanted done to us.

She was diagnosed with non-Hodgkin's lymphoma in the late 1960s when I was about eight. I have no memory of her early years of treatment because in those days, kids and almost everyone else were sheltered from serious illness. We kept on living our enchanted existence: maintaining our busy schedules with school and sports and terrorizing the neighborhood. We were not to notice that Mom lost her hair, no longer could be the den mother, and stopped teaching Sunday school. (I'm not sure if she actually did stop teaching, now that I think of it.) We were not supposed to ask why my sister and I were sent to Dallas to spend the summer with our cousins. Everything was going to be all right. She was going to get better. No need to worry.

The last time I saw Mom, she lay curled in a hospital bed, weighed less than eighty pounds, and could not really speak to say good-bye. A couple of days after that visit, Dad called my brother, sister, and me out of shooting hoops in our driveway with the neighborhood gang to tell us what I think the other kids already knew: Mom had died. She was just short of forty; I was thirteen. In retrospect, I am pretty sure the neighborhood kids had been sent over by their parents to keep us busy and to support us after we heard.

My father was a widower for only a short time. Within six months of our mother's death, short of money but long on optimism, he married his high school sweetheart, who had two kids essentially our ages. We found ourselves transformed from a classic nuclear family to what became a messy, complicated stepfamily.

Not too long afterward, we had our version of "Black Tuesday." The shopping center business grew rapidly, dependent on a major loan that was suddenly called in. Dramatically, seemingly instantly, my father's business collapsed all the way to bankruptcy. Within a few years of our mother dying, our once opulent, carefree existence was over. He had to sell everything at a major loss. To be called to become an oncologist, at least a good one, you usually have a personal family story with cancer. This was mine. I realized that if I were to regain the magic of my childhood and never to have the financial rug pulled out again, I was going to have to build my own future. Dreams of a Broadway career vanished. A career in medicine offered the kind of financial stability I had to have.

The added pressure of a newly merged family made escape attractive, so I went off to boarding school at the Episcopal High School in Alexandria, Virginia. (Coincidentally, Liza, my future wife and co-author, was simultaneously attending the public high school across the street.) In the formal boarding school environment of wearing jackets and ties to everything except sports, surrounded only by boys, complete with a century-old hazing culture, I regained the structured environment that I had lost after my mother's death. I was back on track.

My best friend in high school convinced me to apply to Duke. He said it would be great fun if we went together, but then he bailed on me and went to Williams. In 1979, my father dropped me off at my new and co-ed dorm in Durham, North Carolina, bought me a twelve-pack of beer, gave me a hug and kiss, and drove home. No orientation lectures, no dinner out with the new roommate, no admonishments that I should go to class. With no structure at home and none at college, I was adrift, rudderless, and lost. In a few months, my grades fell. Classes missed. New drugs explored. Any chance at med school slipping away. I had many great friends. I felt utterly alone.

At what turned out to be the lowest point in my life, during my third and final year at Duke—I needed to graduate early to save money—I lay in my bunk in the Sigma Chi fraternity house and prayed out of desperation. I confessed that I had blown my college opportunity. I begged God for divine intervention, even though I had no earthly idea what I meant by that. The next day, as I stood in front of the frat house, tapping the first keg of the evening (as was the job of the social chairman), for the second time in my life, I felt God's shove in the back. I looked up and saw Liza. She was more than beautiful. She was magical, an angel, a "hot" angel. I know this sounds corny, but less than twenty-four hours after they were spoken, I could see that she was the answer to my prayers of the night before. I was in love. We spent the evening together—I got a really good kiss—and I told my fellow Sigma Chis that I had found The Girl. We were almost a caricature of opposites. Liza was the straight-A, church-going, conscientious girl, and I was the dangerous, drug-selling, class-skipping person with no morals. Those who knew both of us were astonished that we had fallen for each other, given our vastly different reputations. But Liza and I knew for sure.

And then, only because of the God-sent Liza, I miraculously redis-covered my calling. I really did want to be a doctor, not just any doctor, but a cancer doctor. I wanted to have an impact, and with Liza's and God's help, I would help transform cancer care. So as soon as she grad-uated, we got married. She went to law school, and I went to medical school. We both secured jobs in Washington, D.C. We bought a house. We had a son and a daughter.

And then Liza got cancer.

CHAPTER 3

Testing

At 2:00 p.m. on Monday, November 20, 2006, I entered a new dimension, a world of strangely noisy machines, unknown words, and unfamiliar tests. I also was barraged with all the familiar elements of healthcare that were once mundane but now seemed more meaningful: doctors, forms, nurses, forms, waiting rooms, forms, needles, and more forms.

John and I headed to Georgetown to start the figuring-out-how-bad-it-is process. John, knowing that I had long been anxious about having an MRI someday, suggested that I take an Ativan. I had the medication on hand to cope with my fear of flying, a problem I had developed after we had children, and I started envisioning what would happen to them if both their parents were killed in a plane crash. Somehow I have always been skilled at imagining how bad things might be, working disasters out to the last mundane detail. Ironically, when it came to my own cancer, I didn't spend a lot of time worrying about how bad it might be or what terrible things would happen. Maybe my expertise in disaster scenarios actually gave me the calm I needed, knowing that no matter what was to come, we would be prepared for it.

After donning a hospital gown and getting an IV for the contrast dye to be injected, I entered the room with the intimidatingly large MRI machine. I had to perform some contortions to position myself on the table facedown and insert my uncovered breasts into two openings on a padded platform. The tech worked hard to ensure that I was as comfortable as possible, bringing me a pillow and a warm blanket. (Did I mention I love the warm blankets in the hospital?) When you already have neck pain, however, lying facedown with your arms over your head for a long time only exacerbates the discomfort. I felt quite alone, with the tech on the other side of a window, speaking to me in a disembodied voice through headphones. Soothed by the Ativan and the local classical music station piped into the headphones, I was able to drift off a bit during the forty-five minutes I was in the machine.

Next, John and I walked to the radiology department for a CT scan of my chest, abdomen, and pelvis to see if there was any evidence of cancer in other parts of my body. One of the radiologists looked at my CT scan while it was being done and said that she did not immediately see anything of concern elsewhere. They would keep watching an indeterminate "something" in my lung, but they weren't particularly concerned about it then. Now we just had to wait until Dr. Willey received the reports, which was going to make for a less than cheery Thanksgiving weekend.

But the day still wasn't over. The kids were at my parents, and we needed to pick them up and tell them…something. We drove mostly in silence. John and I have always been straightforward and honest with our children. There were and still are few secrets among us, and we weren't going to start now. At the same time, we didn't want to frighten them too much. John's profession took some of the terror out of cancer because it was a common dinner-table topic at our house.

They knew, however, that people could die no matter what doctors did or how good they were. Charlie, who was thirteen years old, had been a classmate of Holly Richardson's daughter when Holly developed cancer, so he had seen first-hand the toll that cancer, and particularly breast cancer, takes on a family. In addition, both of our children knew their father had lost his mother to cancer when he was thirteen, so young mothers dying of cancer was a distinct possibility. John and I decided we could tell them only what we actually knew, without any reference to the myriad possibilities. "Mom has breast cancer" seemed an important place to begin. "She is going to have surgery next week. They will remove her right breast, and she'll have chemotherapy after that. It looks as if it isn't anywhere in her body other than her breast. She has good doctors." We decided John would do the talking. I tend to tear up at the slightest provocation, so I probably could not hold it together if I said it out loud to these two expectant and innocent faces I loved.

When we arrived, my parents greeted us at the door, then quickly withdrew to leave us alone and perhaps not to hear us say again that I had cancer. John, Charlie, Emma, and I sat in the family room in the house I grew up in, surrounded by family mementos. John repeated the script we had composed in the car. I struggled not to cry or to look scared, but to portray confidence. I know it was hard for John to say out loud, too, but he is a good actor and an experienced deliverer of bad news, so he pulled it off.

Charlie was in the throes of girls, eighth-grade homework, soccer, baseball, and applications to high schools, so after we finished laying things out, he asked if I was going to be OK. We said we thought so, and he seemed satisfied. I thought Emma, our ten-year-old, was more worried, but she too was ready to move on.

So that was that. John and I had heard terrible news, and we had told our children and my parents a version of that terrible news. It was time to pack up the kids' stuff and thank my parents as profusely as we could in our depleted state for being there for us on a moment's notice. Then the four of us drove home.

John and I got ready for bed and crawled in, searching for a bit of respite from the dramatic changes in our lives since we had gotten out of bed that morning. Instead of reading or watching television as we usually did, we told each other how sorry we were for what was happening to us. We kissed, and we fell asleep. I don't know if John slept, actually, but one of my reactions to great stress is sleeping, and this qualified.

The process of sharing our bad news had only just begun. John and I went to school early the next morning to meet with the head of school and tell him what was going on in our family. He looked surprised but not shocked. After all, he had dealt with this before with Holly. He offered whatever our family might need in the way of support. Then we stopped by our children's home classrooms to let the teachers know and received heartfelt expressions of sympathy, generous offers of help, and assurances of whatever any of us needed.

Having worked our way through the staff, it was my turn to stand in the hallway and tell the other mothers that *I* had breast cancer. It seemed months since pie distribution day, even though it was only the day before. My voice quavered with the shock of saying it out loud, of standing where Holly had stood saying the same thing. And every mother was there because of the traditional pre-Thanksgiving school concert.

The news spread quickly. I didn't even get to tell my very best friend at the school because the word got to her before I could. I couldn't stop myself from telling people; somehow repeating that I had cancer made it more real. Having cancer was going to start affecting my life soon, and I needed to get the facts out before an adult version of the child's game of telephone took things beyond my control. Plus, I tend to wear my heart on my sleeve, so I couldn't *not* tell people. Each reaction was more thoughtful and compassionate than the previous one. Of course, Holly was a ghostly presence. Then I joined my parents in the auditorium for the annual program of a musical number by each grade and each musical group, with sweetness and good cheer overflowing. It was the first time I said to myself, "I'm going to enjoy this moment for what it is because I can and should." And I did.

We spent the day before Thanksgiving at Georgetown for one more test and meetings with doctors. The neck pain I had complained of required a full-body bone scan, which involved more things injected to indicate whether the cancer had metastasized. I wondered if all these foreign substances in my body might give me cancer. (Oh yeah, I already had cancer.) I lay still for a long period as the bone scanner passed slowly over my body. John sat in the small, dark room with me, and we actually joked a bit about things as we watched the machine inch down. Good news! No evidence of cancer in my bones, not even in my neck. John let out a "Woohoo!" I hadn't realized how scared he was about the neck pain and what it might portend. It turned out that I had arthritis in every joint in my body. *Well*, I thought, *let's hope I live long enough for that to be a problem.*

Finally, we went to see Dr. Shawna Willey, the surgical oncologist, to find out what kind of breast cancer I had. I looked around at the other people in the waiting room and wondered if each one was there for a routine mammogram or something more dire. No one looked happy. I know we didn't. Eventually, we were escorted to the examining room. Dr. Willey greeted us both as friends, but she quickly pivoted to her objective physician demeanor, a transition I had seen John perform many times when we were approached by his patients outside the hospital.

Dr. Willey started with the "good" news. She said that the CT did not show any cancer beyond the breast, but she cautioned that a CT cannot show everything. Both the MRI and the CT indicated that there *was* cancer in the breast, but Dr. Willey said that the primary tumor was not really visible on either scan. In fact, she said, even the core needle biopsy did not find a primary tumor. The only evidence of breast cancer from the biopsy was tumor cells in the pieces of my lymphatic system that had been included in the cores, meaning she did not really know exactly where the tumor was in my breast or how big it was. She did know, though, that the tumor was already trying to spread into the rest of my body by way of my lymph system, since that was where they had found cancer cells.

When diagnosed with breast cancer, many women are given a choice between a lumpectomy, in which just the tumor and the area around it are surgically removed in order to conserve as much of the breast as possible, or a mastectomy, in which the entire breast is removed. I was not offered that choice since no one knew precisely where the tumor was located and since we knew the cancer cells had migrated beyond the tumor and throughout the breast. Perhaps that made it easier. Making medical decisions is very hard because the people deciding really cannot know or understand all the potential consequences of each possible choice no matter how well informed they are. I had plenty of difficult choices to come, and I was shell-shocked enough at that point to feel less than competent in determining what I should do.

You'd think being married to an oncologist might help, but John's specialty was gastrointestinal cancers. General community oncologists see all types of cancers and so know a fair bit about each, but in an academic setting, the oncologists are all specialists who know almost everything there is to know about the cancers *they* treat, but not that much about other cancers. John knew that Dr. Willey was a nationally known expert, so he deferred to her. He also deferred to me, recognizing that I was the one who, in the end, would have to live most personally with the decisions and their ramifications.

Perhaps the most important piece of information Dr. Willey had to impart was that my biopsy showed that I had triple-negative breast cancer. I had never heard of this. I knew only that there were estrogen receptors and progesterone receptors, and that you could be positive or negative for those. I asked Dr. Willey to explain triple-negative. She said it meant that my breast cancer did not show positivity for estrogen or progesterone receptors or for the HER-2 protein.

What she did not tell me was that triple-negative was one of the worst kinds of breast cancer. Because its growth is not fueled by hormones, many of the current and more successful drugs are not effective in treating it. In addition, triple-negative breast cancer is relatively rare, comprising only about 10 to 20 percent of all breast cancers, so there was less incentive for researchers to study how best to treat it. It is the most aggressive type and has a poorer prognosis than other forms of breast cancer. Thus, it recurs in about 40 to 50 percent of the cases[1]— which, when I did my own research, was another percentage I didn't like.

1 "Triple-Negative Breast Cancer," www.breastcancer.org/symptoms/diagnosis/ trip_neg, September 9, 2019.

I knew nothing about all of this as Dr. Willey was talking, and I thought that John didn't either. Triple-negative breast cancer was still a fairly new diagnosis at the time, so he was listening intently as well, digesting the information about my diagnosis. He looked worried, and that increased my worry. I needed only to look at them to realize that despite Dr. Willey's upbeat demeanor and tone, my diagnosis was dire.

Dr. Willey then gave an overview of what was to come: surgery, chemotherapy, and radiation. For about a week to ten days after surgery, I would have two tubes from under my arm that would drain fluid away from the area where the breast had been removed to facilitate healing. We would have to empty and measure the drains every twelve hours until the discharge dropped below 10 cc's of fluid. This sounded revolting. I am not a big fan of blood, particularly my own. She prescribed a special bra that I could stuff after surgery that would make it look as if I still had a right breast but that would be soft on my chest. The bra also could hold the bulbs of the drains so the tubes didn't hang loose or catch on anything. Driving was out as long as I had the drains.

In the way your mind works when confronted with life-changing events, I focused on the trivial. I had just bought a stick-shift car, which I loved driving. Would I be able to drive it while I healed from surgery? "No," she replied, an answer that seemed to magnify my despair. But that was only the beginning. She described my future prosthetic breast and the special types of bras I would need with a pocket for the prosthesis and how I could obtain those. She warned me about the possibility of developing lymphedema, a swelling in the arm on the side where the breast has been removed, because of damage to the lymph system that can be caused by breast cancer treatment. She went through a long list of things I wouldn't be able to do with or to my right arm going forward: lift anything over five pounds, get a bug bite or scratch, have a manicure, etc. This sounded nearly impossible. How do you avoid getting a scratch or bug bite on your arm? How do you not lift anything over five pounds? That's hardly any weight at all. The reference is always that a gallon of milk is five pounds. Was just carrying groceries in from the car always going to require help? I began to rebel before we finished the discussion, but I kept it to myself. I was determined to figure out how to work around the restrictions and not get lymphedema.

Without knowing how I was processing all the descriptions of the incredible inconveniences I would face, Dr. Willey moved on to discussing chemotherapy and an option for "neoadjuvant chemo-therapy," which was becoming more widely used in breast cancer. With this approach, a patient receives chemotherapy *before* surgery in the expectation that the treatment will shrink the tumor, allowing the woman more surgical options such as a lumpectomy instead of a mastectomy. Dr. Willey's report from that day said, "My assessment is that she will need a mastectomy, even if we could get a clinical response with chemotherapy, as this tumor has been so difficult to image and identify, and even now assessment as to clinical response would be difficult." Doing chemotherapy first, she told us, meant that it would be difficult to "stage" the cancer—that is, to fully understand how far it had spread. It might change how radiation was done, and it would eliminate the ability to do further study of the tumor, which might give us valuable information about prognosis and treatment choices.

Dr. Claudine Isaacs came down to the breast surgery clinic to join us in her dual roles as an experienced breast oncologist and our good friend. The conversation swirled over my head while John, Dr. Willey, and Claudine talked. I sat in an armchair in a small conference area while the doctors perched on the edges of desks and tables and discussed my case.

John asked some questions that I'm sure were relevant and important, but I really didn't understand a lot of what they were saying. The only thing that seemed clear was that I didn't know enough to make a decision. Dr. Willey noted in her report that I was "understandably eager to get surgery scheduled," so apparently I made it clear that I wanted the breast off my chest as soon as humanly possible. Of all the things I had to be upset about, losing my breast really wasn't one of them. As I mentioned, I wasn't that attached to my breasts. I mean, I was physically attached but not emotionally. Charlie once told me about a T-shirt he saw that said, "Yes, these are fake. My real ones tried to kill me." That was pretty much how I felt.

Because Dr. Willey, Claudine, and John were colleagues and used to discussing what might be the best approach out of the hearing of patients, I think they kind of forgot that this patient was in the room. At the end of their conversation, they looked at me and cheerfully announced, "We have a plan." I was too numb and confused to do more than give a wan smile and stand up. We did have a plan: surgery on the Tuesday after Thanksgiving, six days from now.

No one ever mentioned reconstruction. I spent several years afterward wondering, as I talked to more and more women who had had reconstruction from a mastectomy as part of the original surgery, why this was not one of my options. I resented that I had not been given *that* option or told why it wasn't possible for me. Apparently, everyone had been extremely concerned that the cancer was triple-negative and therefore aggressive. It already had spread to the lymph system, and they wanted me to have a simple, single surgery that would heal quickly so that I could start chemotherapy soon thereafter. In addition, my radiation treatments were likely to affect my breast skin, which could alter the reconstruction in ways that could leave me disfigured.

My next meeting was with Dr. Liu, our choice for my medical oncologist. Our relationship with Claudine made her being my doctor impossible. I knew Minetta from work events, and everyone at Lombardi admired her intellect, thoroughness, caregiving abilities, and thoughtfulness. We greeted each other somewhat morosely. I complained to John later that everybody I knew at Lombardi seemed to look at me with what I called "the mournful oncologist look." They all seemed to know something I didn't, and it frightened me every time I saw it. Minetta's expression was meant as sympathy, of course, but she quickly assumed her professional oncologist demeanor and opened a discussion of my options around chemotherapy, which I would start as soon as I was deemed sufficiently healed from surgery.

She also mentioned neoadjuvant therapy, but I was fairly sure from my discussion with Dr. Willey that I didn't want it. With a difficult-to-pinpoint tumor, I couldn't understand how they would be able to tell what effect the chemotherapy was having. Moreover, the idea of leaving the *known* cancer cells in my body to do God knows what while we were infusing me with chemotherapy that we hoped but didn't *know* would work held no appeal. Minetta supported my preference for the traditional surgery and then chemotherapy route. She explained the chemo protocols, the regular blood tests to see how my body was handling the chemo, and then, if all was well, my treatment. She went over the possible side effects of the various drugs and some clinical trials that I might join. I was to follow up with her in an office visit after surgery to get the full "new oncology patient" workup and discussion, which was good because I was exhausted and no longer processing much.

I just prayed that the decisions I had made were the ones that were going to lead to a complete cure. I fantasized about spraying Raid down my throat to kill the cancer cells floating in my body. After this onslaught of information and decisions, returning home that night and getting organized for our Thanksgiving dinner the next day seemed almost a relief. The kids were delighted to be out of school, and looking around at them, at John, at our home, reminded me to feel some gratitude, even in the midst of a catastrophe.

CHAPTER 4

Seeing Signs

The most basic encounter with a patient is called a "history and physical," or H&P. It is purposefully standardized, balancing comprehensiveness with efficiency. First, we extract the patient's details, focused on the most immediate complaints, medical history, active medicines, who's their daddy, smoking, exercise, and so on. Then we do a physical exam, flashing our stethoscope so that we look the part, and finishing off with a discussion of what we think and recommend.

Fundamental to this process are the symptoms and signs of common diagnoses. Symptoms are clues provided by the patient, individual pieces of a thousand-piece puzzle. Some pieces help solve the ultimate diagnosis puzzle, while some have nothing to do with the puzzle at all, a distraction accidentally thrown into the wrong box, never to fit no matter how hard you push. Many symptoms lead to doctors ordering tests that go nowhere. Many are incorrectly put aside for later, much to the joy of tort attorneys. Hoping not to miss even the smallest clue, we urge the patient to tell us everything.

We are taught to start fresh with every patient encounter: Don't assume things are the same as before, and don't miss any new detail. Dutifully, I go into an examining room where a longtime patient of mine with stomach cancer is waiting for a routine follow-up. After brief social exchanges, I ask, "How are you?" In this context, it is not a formality but a purposeful start to the H&P questions. Out pours the list of problems, neatly written on the spiral notepad pulled from his breast pocket. "My stomach hurts, I am short of breath, I lost some weight, I am having trouble walking, and not sure but it feels like there's this lump on my rib, and it hurts when I poke at it."

Now *that* is a list! Where do I even start? I have another patient waiting next door, and at 9:30 in the morning I already am running late, so efficiency and speed are of the essence. Is this impressive list of symptoms related to one problem or several? How many puzzles are we dealing with? Are the symptoms new or old? Is my patient's rib pain a metastasis from his stomach cancer or simply tenderness from poking it so much? Is his shortness of breath a small blood clot in his lungs or anxiety? We go through everything, including his recent diet, any new exercise, new meds, looking for anything—please let this be something *other* than recurrent cancer—that could explain his symptoms. After exhausting all lines of questioning, after not being 100 percent sure that his rib pain is "nothing," I arrange for a CT scan that day. Outwardly calm, he heads to radiology. He knows to contact me as soon as the test is done. At end of clinic, I see his e-mail. Curious and nervous myself, I swing by radiology to review the scan. Thank God, the scan is negative, and labs were fine. It does not look to be cancer.

An easy short e-mail back: "…exhale, scan fine, labs fine. Take some antacid for a few days and quit poking your ribs. See you in 6 mo."

Some patients, the know-it-alls or KIAs, have assessed their symptoms and announce the diagnosis with the recommended treatment protocol they found on Google. Our role is limited to confirming their diagnosis and treatment plan, expressing our gratitude and awe at their brilliance, and providing the prescription. (And BTW, could we phone that in?) Eventually, I may be replaced by a process where you can enter your symptoms into the app on your phone, drive to the pickup window at the local CVS on the way home from teleworking at the nearby Starbucks, scan the Aetna insurance/diagnosis bar code supplied to confirm it is indeed you, double-check with the retina scan, and get your prescription. Better still, a drone will deliver the drugs. No gowns, no probing, and definitely no human contact.

As with my stomach cancer patient, after engaging in the laborious process of connecting the dots of a seemingly random collection of patient-provided complaints, we put together a "differential diagnosis," a list of most likely diagnoses with our best guess of what is wrong. We confirm and refine our list after a physical exam. We either make the diagnosis, do tests to confirm, or both. Then we treat.

Signs are much easier. They are objective and part of the physical exam; they are yes or no. In medical school, we learn signs from texts and lectures, but when you actually uncover one yourself, the pathognomonic finding staring back at you, it is literally breathtaking, hard to refrain from gasping out loud in front of the patient with a "eureka." Signs are like big pieces of a toddler's wooden puzzle. With only one piece in hand depicting a pair of giraffes from Noah's Ark, you know pretty much for certain that the firm, enlarged lymph node right above the left clavicle of my stomach cancer patient—a Virchow's node—is a death sentence. No other tests needed, just basic observations. Signs do not require interpretation; some do not even require follow-up testing. However, just as with a religious experience, in order to see a sign, you have to be looking for one.

Liza and I were getting dressed one morning. I was brushing my teeth, and Liza was just out of the shower, without clothes, bending over the sink looking in the mirror. I happened to look at her breasts as she leaned forward. There, without my really looking for it, was the sign. Her right breast was not "right." When she leaned forward, the skin dimpled a bit, tethered by something below the surface. Very few things could cause this, a short differential diagnosis list. This was almost certainly breast cancer. And when it involves the skin, also known as inflammatory breast cancer, it is almost always fatal. A one-piece puzzle.

I said nothing. I somehow swallowed my eureka gasp.

I did not want to upset her. My telling her would not help anything. Sure, I am a pro at sharing bad news, explaining complex concepts in simple, understandable ways. I love her, and we are the perfect couple. This should be my job. She hates to not know something. I should tell her. And yet I didn't. After all, I saw her breast tissue dimpling out of the corner of my eye. Maybe I did not see things correctly. I might have remembered the wrong sign. As we went through the morning routine, with breakfast, the sports page, the quick schedule rundown, the image of her dimpled breast invaded my every thought.

It's not as if Liza hadn't sensed something going on with that breast. She mentioned that it felt odd, as if it were swollen. She went to see Shawna Willey, who was the lead person on her breast team at Georgetown. They took her history, did a physical exam of her breasts, but could not replicate the tethering of her breast on leaning forward. The sign was gone. The mammogram did not show anything. "God, please let me have been wrong."

Shawna said, "Let's get a biopsy to be sure."

As part of this biopsy, Liza was approached to be part of a clinical trial. The trial involved allowing our researchers to study her biopsy sample. In breast cancer, there is a study for everything: Remember, researchers go where the money is. As studies go, the one Liza participated in was easy, with no added risk, but no added benefit. When we found out that her biopsy was benign, a sample would be banked with other benign breast biopsy samples to study as a group at some future point. Our friend and my colleague, Dr. Minetta Liu, was in charge of the study, and of course, Liza signed the consent form. Little did we suspect there would be more consents, more chances to contribute to science.

Biopsies take a week or more to report out. We went on with life. Even though I was extremely worried that she had inflammatory breast cancer, I had weirdly forgotten she already had a biopsy: I am skilled at compartmentalizing. I don't remember our discussing it. I really did not want to talk about it as I would have to mention what I saw and what it probably meant. If I was right, I was determined that someone else would tell her the news.

My least favorite part of my job is giving bad news. It could be a bad scan showing that the cancer is back, and death is certain. It could be that we have no more treatment options, hope is running dry, and it's time for hospice. The worst for me, fortunately rare as some other poor doctor typically has broken the bad news, is to tell someone who is praying with all their might that the biopsy was benign that, in fact, it was malignant. For many, I will deliver the worst news they will ever hear.

First, you see the patient's eyes go blank, their thoughts sunk deep inside, no longer hearing what you are saying. Finally, recognizing my failure to communicate, I stop talking altogether, waiting for the patient to resurface. After a minute or two, the eyes clear, and the patient is back—shocked, full of disbelief and questions. Tears appear, and the patient is afraid even to glance at the spouse. The spouse is doing everything to be strong. Simultaneously, they get brave enough to look at each other. You see life-changing shock, pain, fear, sadness, denial. For sure, I did not want to be the messenger, but even more, I really did not want to look Liza in the eye.

Out of necessity, I am a creature of habit. To maintain all the moving parts of a busy cancer practice and research career, I set aside time first thing after I arrive at the office every day to stop, review, and organize. I am focused, awake, clear, and undistracted. In 2006, electronic medical records were not so ubiquitous, and CT scans, biopsy results, letters from other docs, and orders to sign came to me by fax or mail. I would flip through the new stack: last night's faxes, the end-of-the-day dump that I didn't review the night before. I efficiently sort through the reports, sign off on any orders, review my schedule for the day, and treat myself to my one cup of doctor's lounge coffee. Once done, it's showtime!

I am supposed to receive results only on my patients. Getting records on other doctors' patients is technically a privacy HIPAA violation. But on this particular Monday, I came across a pathology report positive for breast cancer. I don't do breast cancer. I looked down to the bottom. There was my name. For some reason, I had been copied to receive the report. I looked at the top for the name of the patient. My heart stopped. The image of Liza's dimpled breast returned. I looked again at the path report, the name, the summary diagnosis. There must be a mistake.

Aside from an occasional antibiotic script on a Sunday afternoon, a quick look at a rash, a funny mole, recommendations on which cold medicine to buy, doctors are never supposed to treat family. I'm shocked when I hear that my colleagues are not only their spouse's primary doctor but also treating themselves. I am not sure if I hesitated. I knew all the rules: I should not be telling Liza that she has cancer. This is for a professional to do—her doctor's job, not mine. And yet I picked up the phone and called. She answered. "You have breast cancer," I said. "The biopsy is positive."

I have no memory of what Liza said next. She will tell you I have no memory of anything she has ever said…. We were both in a state of shock. I could not think straight. My mind was racing. This was retribution for my long disparagement of the breast cancer machine. The breast cancer world hates me. I could just imagine the smug faces mocking me for trying to undermine the success of breast cancer research. I am pretty sure that while my mind was flying from one "end of days" image to the next, Liza and I actually were talking to each other. I was answering her questions as best I could. We were already in planning mode. What is next? Who do we need to see? How fast can that happen? What do we need to cancel? Thanksgiving was approaching—what did we need to organize for that? We need to move quickly.

My wife had inflammatory breast cancer. My world as I knew it was over. And I was the messenger who delivered the diagnosis. Thankfully, having broken a major unwritten rule of medicine by delivering the dire news by phone, I did not have to see her eyes.

Then, as if from heaven, Minetta Liu walked into my office. As the head of the biopsy trial, Minetta also had the path report faxed to her. She was shocked at what she found, dropped everything, came to my office, and found us there on the phone. She took the phone from me. At that moment, Minetta officially relieved me of my role as the physician and messenger—maybe my shortest doctor-patient relationship ever. At that moment, I assumed my new role, which felt like a promotion: I was going to be Liza's caregiver.

In my practice, I used my emotional armor to protect myself against feeling the pain I was inflicting. Coping with the diagnosis I was giving was their problem, not mine. I needed to teach them about the disease, develop the plan of attack, and organize the next steps. I needed to stay objective and above the emotion. After that split second on the telephone with my wife, I lost my armor. I now felt what my patients were feeling. I wasn't capable of hearing anything anyone had to say until I had recovered from the shock. Best to just wait, sit and wait.

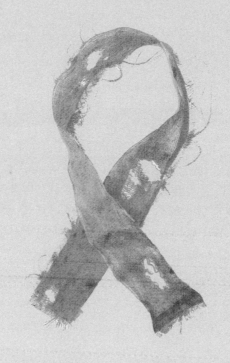

PART 2

WHAM

Cancer 101

New Research Building Auditorium

Lombardi Comprehensive Cancer Center

Georgetown University

Washington, D.C.

May 2010

O*n behalf of Georgetown University and our cancer center team, let me welcome you to this week's Mini-Med School lecture. We have only two hours to cover one of the biggest topics in medicine and research today, so we will need to stay high level, big picture. But I hope you will leave with a better understanding both of the diseases we call cancer and the work ahead as we seek to find cures.*

Let's start with a basic question: Who gets cancer? We all know the usual suspects. Certainly smokers, drinkers, red meat eaters, fornicators, sunbathers, couch potatoes, non-God-fearing people. But you must recognize that most smokers, drinkers, fornicators, sunbathers, couch potatoes, non-God-fearing people don't actually get cancer. Why, as we smugly eat nothing but cardboard, spend our weekends running marathons, while walking our dogs and engaging in a clean-living, sunblock-wearing, God-fearing existence, do we get cancer?

The current wisdom is that all of us get cancer, likely many times over our lives. It would not surprise me if we discover that some of us have daily bouts. OK, now I have your attention! If true, then this raises the important question: Why do some people die of cancer while some never knew they had it in the first place? Is it all just bad luck, or do we have some control over our destiny?

It is truly a miracle that we each evolve (if you still believe in evolution) from a primordial glob of cells in our mother's womb into an elegantly arranged, complex being. Step by step, our original undifferentiated cells begin to take on their assigned roles. Cells that will become your GI tract activate a set of DNA-coded programs that allow them to migrate to the right place, forming the feeding and sewer system tube that runs through us. Some cells arrogantly march off to become our brains (of course, they think they are better than the others). Each cell migrates to get in the right place and assumes its assigned role. Each cell still has all the information to do all the things the other cells can do, but once differentiated, the now-unused sections of the DNA go quiet, unnecessary, and obsolete.

And then, life happens. Our cells are under constant attack from external forces that can damage DNA. Spoiler alert: The following discussion will make you afraid to eat, breathe, go outside, kiss someone, or have a stiff drink—all of which you will certainly need and, as your physician this evening, I will prescribe right now. Everything we do as humans, and I mean everything, puts our cells to work. And the more work our cells have to do, the more chance for error.

Most of the time, our cells can repair the potholes of life and get back to normal. Sometimes the damage to the DNA is so egregious that the new cell raises the white flag and sets off a program called apoptosis, essentially dismantling and—being very environmentally responsible—reusing the cell's parts to make a new one. In many ways, traditional chemo takes advantage of this cellular recycling, intentionally damaging the DNA of the cancer cells beyond repair in the hopes of activating the apoptosis machinery to break those suckers down for parts. But sometimes the broken DNA slips under the radar. This new clone is now different from your original set, having acquired new and sometimes life-threatening functions. The new cells can lose their ability to control themselves; one program within the DNA stops working while another previously silenced part of the code is reawakened, now uncontrolled, stuck in the "on" position. The new clones divide unchecked; they somehow reboot the genes allowing travel to other parts of the body. Interfering with normal organ function, they continue to divide and spread and overwhelm anything in their paths…until they kill you. Or until chemo intervenes. Cancer cells need to divide more than our normal cells, so traditional chemo was designed to kill cancer cells more than normal cells. Except when it doesn't.

Chemo damages DNA in a brutally non-specific way and, while chemo has cured many people, it often leaves behind a great deal of collateral damage to normal cells. Newer targeted therapies for cancer are designed to fix broken molecular switches in a much more precise, smart-bomb approach. We can now determine which switches are stuck on and can turn them back off using new, pretty cool drugs. These new agents have made a dramatic impact both in improvements in effectiveness and in reductions in side effects, less collateral damage. Most of our hottest research today involves uncovering each patient's cancer genetic makeup, defining what is actually broken in their tumor's DNA, and administering the right drug for that patient's particular cancer. We all hope to continue our shift away from our current imprecise, side-effect-laden drugs and replace them with what we now call precision medicine.

Moving on. True or false: A cancer patient's immune system is in some way broken, and that is why they got cancer. OK, show of hands, how many say true? Well over half say that is true. And false? Very few hands this time. How many fall into the "I don't know" category? OK, you people are the honest ones. It turns out "I don't know" actually might be the right answer! Let's take a look at our understanding of the role of the immune system on cancer as we start 2010.

First, the immune system is elegantly designed to seek out and destroy foreign invaders such as bacteria, viruses, a splinter in a finger, and, of course, a donor organ that was transplanted. It does this by detecting foreign proteins and activating a cascade of events that mobilize a literal army of cells designed to destroy the foreign invader. You might logically ask why we would think our immune system would "see" our cancers. After all, cancer is made up of our own cells, not alien invaders. The answer? Remember those mutations we just talked about? It turns out that when the DNA is mutated, it often produces a totally new protein, one that the person's immune system has never seen before. So, in theory, a cancer cell should be detected by the immune system that should be able to attack and remove it.

I was lucky to be trained by some of the real pioneers in cancer immune therapy and have devoted much of my academic research career to figuring out how our fascinating immune system could help in the fight against cancer. My particular angle is vaccines, yes, vaccines, that could help stimulate the immune system to recognize and kill cancer. At this point, mainstream cancer scientists think we immune therapy geeks are barking up the wrong tree. They feel that harnessing the immune system will play little role in treating cancer. Sure, they acknowledge the limited but real impact that interferon—which scored a Time magazine cover— and IL-2 have had in kidney cancers and melanomas. These drugs work by revving up the existing immune response to a higher level. While these treatments come with a lot of serious side effects, we clearly see some patients experience a dramatic reduction in their cancers and some patients seemingly cured. These amazing responses in these few patients are proof the immune system can work. We immune therapy geeks just need to figure out how.

At our cancer meetings, held in convention centers big enough to host a tractor pull, our sparsely attended science sessions on immune therapy or vaccines have been stuck in small rooms tucked in back corridors. In contrast, chemotherapy sessions are in rooms so large they have their own weather. Are we discouraged? Yes. Our grants remain unfunded because traditional research reviewers say we are crazy. The last grant I wrote was rejected three times because the reviewers were sure that nothing would come of our new idea to combine vaccines—which we clearly showed could dial up the immune cells against GI cancer—with new drugs called checkpoint inhibitors. Instead of adding fuel to the immune engine, these new drugs are designed to cut the brakes. Some researchers have shown that cancer often blocks the oncoming army of immune cells, and we believe these drugs would prevent that from happening. Then the immune system would be free to do its thing and kill the cancer. Our reviewers at the NCI did not agree. What some see as innovative, others see as crazy.

But if we are right, it is logical to assume that each of us gets cancer all the time, and that most of the time, our immune system does its job. It is only when the immune system fails to detect the cancer or when the immune system is prevented from doing its job that cancers grow and threaten our lives.

If it is really all about our immune system, cancer prevention advocates should stop blaming red meat and booze and other joys of life. Maybe we should urge bolstering our immune system through lifelong training. But how? It's actually simple: Expose it to stuff. Vaccines, of course, but also viruses, bacteria, dirt, fingernails, someone else's germs, pollen, peanut butter, dogs, cats, horses, dust mite feces, insect venom, poison ivy, and dairy. Every time our immune system detects something strange and foreign, it is distinguishing between self and non-self, dangerous and not so dangerous. While we know a lot about this, there is even more we do not know. Why are some of us are super-sensitive to certain things and develop life-threatening immune "over-response" *allergic reactions, while others can do or ingest anything with no issues? One theory has to do with our microbiome.*

Our microbiome is part of us—it might actually be the location of our souls. We are all covered, inside and out, with billions of bacteria. Why would we have evolved over millions of years retaining all these stinky bacteria if it were not only useful but also critical to our health? There is more bacterial DNA in our skin, our mouths, and our colons than human DNA. I consider the microbiome as our own, personal coral reef. In health, it's perfectly balanced, a thing of beauty, functioning in harmony with itself and with us. But when out of balance, from antibiotics, poor nutrition, or my favorite, inadequate consumption of dirt, we whitewash the coral reef. Bad bacteria take over, and illness ensues. My guess is many answers will emerge as we explore this new world. But let's face it, if the National Cancer Institute was not going to fund grants on immune system research, the agency is unlikely to fund a study of poop.

Speaking of our GI tracts, here's another question; Can you eat your way out of cancer? The snacks we have for you tonight are "healthy," veggies, low-fat cheese, low-salt crackers, juice, water. But is this really healthier than a few cookies and a glass of wine? I am always struck by the fact that after a patient has cancer, he or she feels compelled to dramatically modify behavior, especially when it comes to food: no red meat, turmeric in everything, lots of ginger, green tea, selenium, huge doses of vitamins, no more coffee unless consumed through an enema (not kidding), and the list goes on. Why is one person absolutely sure that eating garlic with every meal will cure cancer and the next is equally convinced that a combination of high dose IV vitamin C and smoking marijuana is the answer? Completely rational, highly educated people who challenge everything, who would never change their life choices and behaviors before they got cancer, now alter everything based on an e-mail sent by their crazy uncle who is sure that eating raw fungus was how his friend's cancer was cured.

The reality is that we don't know how diet alters our health, and you should question anyone who says otherwise. Certainly, some foods and diets are harder on us and might cause more mutations than other foods. Generally, I'm a fan of the so-called Mediterranean diet, not too much meat, more fruits and vegetables. But maybe more important, stop smoking, get sleep, exercise as much as you can, be the right weight. Booze is OK, but not too much. Beyond these recommendations, your guess is as good as mine. The most important advice I give is, "Don't forget to live."

I start almost every new patient visit addressing the "why me" question. While it is true that bad behaviors increase our risk of getting cancer—almost all of my patients never did anything wrong, at least not on a regular basis. My patients are mostly wonky Washingtonians, marathon-running, cardboard-eating people who somehow got cancer. If we continue to cling to this doing-something-wrong paradigm, figuring out cancer causality becomes impossible. All patients need some answer on which to blame their diagnosis, something they can tell family and friends. The reality is that despite all the research, we really don't understand why some people get cancer, and some do not. I think a lot of cancer is actually random. The manager gene is taken out randomly and...WHAM. Or our immune system fails to recognize the cancer as foreign and...WHAM. We can increase our chances of getting cancer by gambling more often with behaviors that beat up the DNA, but even church-going, homeless-helping, marathon-running, cardboard-eating people get cancer.

In fact, even the wife of an oncologist.

CHAPTER 5

Knowing Too Much

In the first few weeks after Liza's diagnosis, we saw a lot of doctors, nearly all colleagues, some close friends. I tried to maintain my practice and my other hospital duties, never actually taking formal time off. Since Liza was being treated at Georgetown, I usually would meet her in a waiting room, sometimes forgetting to take off my white coat, which provoked inquisitive stares from the other patients. On a couple of occasions, we sat alongside my patients, small talk awkwardly drifting to either their cancer issues or Liza's.

During one of Liza's scans, I sat in the waiting room next to one of my patients and his wife. After my patient went back for his test, his wife started sharing her family's experiences. She asked how Liza was doing and how I was doing. As we talked, our relationship transformed from one of doctor and patient to peers. She offered useful insights, tips from a much more experienced caregiver. A part of me welcomed this inter-action, but a part was unsettled, feeling my objectivity wall crumbling a bit. To avoid these encounters in the future, when Liza was getting a test or an infusion, I would go back to my office, do a few e-mails, make a few calls, or host a meeting. She would call when done. Sometimes we met to debrief; sometimes she would say she was fine and go home. I did stay through most doctor's meetings, taking notes, listening to the plans, and trying to figure out what was going on.

Wherever two or more are gathered, I cannot keep my mouth shut. If an idea pops into my head, I express it. I have gotten better at not stepping in when others are talking, but I am not perfect even with significant effort. I tried hard just to listen to Liza's doctors, but I interrupted all the time. I asked questions, I clarified, I reworded what they had said to make sure that we both understood. (Today this is called *mansplaining*.) Since I'm incredibly impatient, when I needed the discussion to move forward a few tracks, I would interrupt in doctor language, direct the discussion toward its conclusion, and skip the parts that I already knew, even though this might leave Liza behind. I urgently needed to understand the punch line. Figuring out how we were going to beat this thing kept my mind from wandering to a bad place.

I was in medical limbo: discussing strategies with Liza's doctors and being determined not to direct her treatment. I could see trust in Liza's eyes, but I also saw fear and vulnerability. She looked lost. I could have exerted my paternalistic oversight of her care, and she might have welcomed it, but I could not. This was her life, her body. My knowledge was useful to collect the information and ensure that Liza understood the details as best she could. She needed to know what she was buying. And yet I was hardly like the other husbands taking notes in my clinic. I already knew what we were being told—and I knew it wasn't good. The notes I took were for Liza; it was going to be *her* decision, not *ours*. I played the spousal role and served as her sounding board, offering to re-explain what we had been told, responding to additional questions that Liza had. Somehow I remained coolly objective, maintaining my traditional doctor distance with Liza as we discussed her options. As I do with all my patients in virtually all clinical scenarios, I had opinions and preferences for Liza's treatments. I knew what I would do if it had been *me* with the cancer. When patients ask me, "What would you do if it were your wife?" I immediately change the question to "What would I do if it were *me*?" That I know how to answer. Treatment preferences are very difficult to make for someone else. When it came time for Liza to make the final choices, I stayed on the sidelines.

The year 2006 was my thirteenth year of practice. I had cared for about 2,500 cancer patients. Many were cured, but because my practice often involved being the doctor of last resort, upward of 70 percent had died—more than 1,700 people. I thought I had seen it all. I knew how to deal with high-risk cancer. I knew how to read patients and families, giving them the information they needed but not sharing what *could* happen, what dying of cancer looks like. Not until I really had to. Until then, I would stick to the positive, focus on how we were going to beat this thing.

Which of the 2,500 patients can I remember? Surprisingly for a guy who cannot remember his children's names, I remember many. But the ones who are seared into the little gray cells, the ones who visit when I cannot sleep at night, are the young ones who died too soon, whose cancers came out of nowhere. The ones like Liza.

Liza had a bad cancer, maybe curable, but in no way was this certain. In 2006, triple-negative breast cancer was a relatively new sub-classification, but we did know a few frightening characteristics. It was more aggressive, less responsive to treatment, and more likely fatal. We had not caught it early despite intensive efforts to do so. It came out of nowhere, grew quickly, spread to nodes. It had invaded her ducts and lymph channels near the skin, just shy of what we call inflammatory breast cancer, a terrible, ominous progression so fast and invasive that cancer cells almost certainly have spread throughout her body. True inflammatory breast cancer is nearly always fatal. This was a raging cancer. We were panicked. Time mattered.

My mind constantly strayed to the possibility that Liza actually could die from this. In fact, she could die from this within a few years. Sure, surgery cures some people, but a cancer like this? Almost certainly cancer cells were running around her body, looking for a new home: liver, lung, her amazing brain. We had come upon our first major decision—should we "pull the root" and do surgery first, or start with chemo and then do surgery?

I wanted to get the damn thing off her body, surgery asap. Minetta mentioned a trial where chemo is given first, before surgery—"neo-adjuvant" we cancer docs call it. Minetta did not push this option, but it was clear she liked it. Maybe she would have pushed it harder if we were among her regular patients. I still wonder what she would have said if I had asked what she would have done in Liza's shoes. The neo-adjuvant strategy has since become a new standard of care, and it's almost certainly the way Liza would have been treated now. In fact, we were offered a clinical trial that would turn out to be quite positive. Too afraid of this new approach, panicked to get the cancer that was growing in front of our eyes off her chest, we declined the only trial we were offered that, in the end, was actually positive.

Shawna Willey said that even if Liza did respond well to the chemo, it would not save her breast, which was coming off either way. What if the chemo did not work? In my imagination, reinforced with the personal experience of too many patients with similar consequences, I could see only that the cancer would grow, grab onto her ribs and chest wall, and never be removed. Necrotic, foul-smelling, dying, infected tissue eating away at her chest wall would be a terrible way to die and a vision too traumatic to share with anyone.

We did not discuss the decision for long. Shawna was leaning toward surgery: Minetta if anything was leaning toward chemo first. We ran it by Claudine, who deferred to us. We had an operating room date scheduled, and a change to a chemo-first strategy would require a new set of tests, appointments, and likely further delays in getting started. It was decided to pull the rapidly invading weed as soon as possible, see how bad it really was, and know for sure. We can treat the yard later.

The surgery was scheduled for a week later. Any time lag between the decision to do something and actually doing it is excruciating. What do you mean waiting a week? JUST ONE MINUTE AGO we discussed how aggressive this cancer is, and now we are going to let it grow for a week and do nothing? You could almost hear the snap, crackle, and pop of the growing and dividing cells as we lay in bed at night. It was a very long week.

We made love two nights before the surgery—we are planners, you know. It was not joyful. It was warm and soft, but mostly sad and quiet. We knew this night was going to be the last time Liza would have two breasts, although that point went completely unspoken. I wanted to remember what she looked like and form a lasting memory. I would have taken a picture. For once, I knew better than even to ask. (It is a shame that we never had taken somewhat spicy pictures when we were younger.) Even that night, Liza did not want any touching or pressure on her breast. We did not ever really talk about the impact of her surgery on our sex life and our marriage. What was there to talk about? A mastectomy had to happen. The first priority was to live; we will figure out our sex life later. Frankly, to this day we rarely have discussed her treatment's impact on our sex life, and even then, only tangentially and uncomfortably. On that night, I knew it would not be the same again. Not necessarily bad, just not the same. I am not that much of a "breast guy" anyway. I would survive. It was not about me; it was not my breast. I was sad, scared, angry, and resentful. Bottling up one's feelings turns out to disrupt sleep.

CHAPTER 6

And Away We Go

I t was the day before surgery. We had managed to go through the motions of a normal weekend: a play at the Shakespeare Theatre on Friday night, a football game on Sunday. I had managed to keep the enormous implications of my diagnosis at bay for the most part, although occasionally I would be shaken by visions of my body cut open, my breast removed, my arms punctured with needles, my hair gone. And now it was Monday. The children were back in school, and I had to have one more procedure—as it turned out, the most painful one of all—the purpose of which was to identify a sentinel node.

John and I made our way to the nuclear medicine department, where a medical technician made three injections of a tracer material into my right breast around the areola. The material was designed to determine if the cancer had made it into the lymph nodes under my arm. It goes to the first lymph node into which the lymphatic fluid from the breast drains, the sentinel node, so the surgeon can see which one to remove to examine for evidence of cancer. The pathologist then quickly examines the sentinel node while the patient is still in surgery, and if he or she finds cancer cells in the lymph node, the surgeon then removes all the underarm or axillary lymph nodes.[1] My breast was still black and blue from the core needle biopsy and my failure to follow post-procedure instructions, so maybe that made it worse, but it was still a needle stuck into one's breast just around the nipple area. All the pain and discomfort were in pursuit of keeping me alive, so I didn't complain, aside from vigorous writhing.

John actually seemed rather shaken by my visible and audible distress. Concerned and vicarious in anguish, he tentatively checked to make sure I was all right to go on alone. He headed back to the cancer center as I went on to my pre-surgery checkup. There a nurse would determine if I was healthy enough to undergo surgery and if accommodations needed to be made by the surgeon and anesthesiologist to ensure that I survived, both physically and cognitively. Still disturbed by the nuclear medicine experience, I also was preoccupied with all the logistics necessary to cover the rest of my life while I was out of commission. How were the kids going to get where they needed to be each day? I had to excuse myself from various jobs and figure out how the dog was going to be fed and walked, and so on. The feeling that there were loose ends yet to be tied up lingered when I arrived at the pre-op office to meet with a nurse. She asked me to list my medications, gave me an EKG, instructed me how to wash myself properly before surgery ("Dial soap only"), and told me to be sure to use clean sheets and nightclothes. Hurray, I got to add laundry *and* changing sheets to my to-do list. Then she took my blood pressure.

"Your blood pressure is high," she said.

"I see that," I sighed.

---

1 "Sentinel Node Biopsy," www.mayoclinic.org/tests-procedures/sentinel-node-biopsy/about/pac-2085264, September 7, 2019.

"You should try to reduce the stress in your life," she admonished me.

Reduce the stress in my life? I'm forty-three years old, I have two children, I have just been diagnosed with the worst possible breast cancer, I'm having one of my breasts removed tomorrow, and you just gave me a list of more things to do between now and tomorrow morning. In a way I was grateful; she reminded me that I still could laugh at something, albeit bitterly.

That night we had a routine family dinner, made non-routine by going over the plans with the kids about what was going to happen in the morning, who was going to take them to school, who was going to pick them up, how they would get to their after-school activities, and so on. We tried to make light of what was coming. I'm sure there were jokes about there being less of me when I came home.

After we got the kids to bed, I got into bed, turned off the light, and finally broke down. I was scared about undergoing the surgery and dying under anesthesia or getting some terrible infection. I was afraid of the pain, the drains. Finally, I was allowing myself to grieve the loss of my breast and imagining how I would look and what it might mean for our sex life. The night before, John and I had sex for the last time with both of my breasts intact. We were very aware of that but didn't really discuss the possible effect of my being without one. I would look deformed, asymmetrical, and scarred. My breasts were an important part of our sex life. I liked to be touched and kissed and caressed there, and John clearly enjoyed doing those things. Would I still enjoy sex without a breast? Would John find me too altered to enjoy sex with me anymore?

On the 2019 Netflix show *Dead to Me*, the main character, Jen Harding, has had a double mastectomy due to having the BRCA gene. The character, played by Christina Applegate, who herself had a double mastectomy because of her genetic makeup, confides to her friend that her husband had stopped even touching her after her mastectomy because he was disgusted by her. I'm sure many women wonder if that could happen to them, and I worried that John would be repulsed by me. He is a generous and nonjudgmental person, and—another advantage of being married to an oncologist—he has seen plenty of people with body-altering surgery. But his relationship with his patients was quite different from that with his wife and sexual partner. Their attractiveness wasn't going to be his problem, but maybe mine was. I could only hope that we would find a way to go on in the bedroom.

I sobbed in the dark while John held me, acknowledging my fear and my grief, assuring me as best he could that I was, and we were, going to be all right. Finally, I cried myself out and fell asleep. I am not sure that John was able to sleep at all.

We were up very early the next morning so I could comply with the instructions about showering and arriving at the hospital two hours ahead of my nine o'clock surgery time. I put a few things in a bag and dressed in sweatpants and a top that opened in front as I would not be able to put anything over my head for a while. John ate some breakfast while I dutifully let nothing pass my mouth. I fed the dog and glanced at the newspaper. I kissed the sleeping children good-bye, hoping it wouldn't be forever.

After checking in with the Surgery Center at Georgetown, we were called back to an area with curtained areas around gurneys. The nurse smiled warmly at me as she gave instructions about undressing and packing up my things to be sure they went to my room later. I began to cry again as I wandered around removing my clothes, taking my two-cupped bra off for the last time. I somehow ended up being assigned to a pre-surgery cubicle that did not have a bed in it. Instead,

I got a chair. I settled into the chair while tears trickled down my face. I had lost my brave face at some point during the preceding afternoon.

Dr. Willey arrived and greeted me cheerfully. I went through giving my name, my birthdate, and what surgery I was having on what body part for the umpteenth time. The anesthesiologist then came in and went through his set of questions about dentures, loose teeth, and previous experiences with anesthesia. Then he told me about his use of nerve blocks in these types of surgery, which they were finding reduced post-operative pain and led to fewer post-anesthesia complications. I was delighted to hear that, at least in one way, maybe things wouldn't be quite as bad as I had expected. The anesthesiology resident got my IV started (Hurray, another needle!), and the hour of my mastectomy approached.

Finally, the anesthesiologist and the surgery resident came to escort me to the operating room. John gave me a kiss and scurried upstairs to get a bit of work done. In one of the more surreal parts of my breast cancer experience, because I was not on a gurney, I walked with the two doctors down the hall and into the operating room, as they carried my IV bags and instructed me to pick up a hair net on the way in. I crawled up on the operating table and settled in for a long winter's nap. In retrospect, perhaps the unorthodox entry to the OR was a useful, even amusing, distraction.

After I arranged myself on the metal operating table, a nurse put a canula tube around my head so I could get some oxygen through my nose. I was jolted as the cold air blew up my nostrils. Then someone placed a mask over my face. I was out.

* * *

The next thing I remember was awaking groggily in a small curtained area, lying in a bed with John sitting nearby. It always takes me a bit to come out of anesthesia, but I was relieved not to feel nauseated. I was also thankful to be alive and not in pain. Three hours had passed since I went under. The big question was what they had found.

Dr. Willey quickly appeared at my bedside. She informed me that the sentinel node had been found to have cancer in it, and thus they had had to remove my axillary lymph nodes in an attempt to stop its spread into the rest of my body. I might have been groggy, but I remembered that this could mean I had cancer in *all* the nodes like Holly, and that was going to be very bad news.

I don't understand why doctors give you important information just when you are coming out of anesthesia. I rarely can remember anything after my colonoscopy, and yet every time the doctor appears at my bedside as soon as I have awoken. This time I had John there. He, of course, remembered and understood everything Dr. Willey said. He had to recite it to me repeatedly over the next few days and weeks as I tried to understand what they had found and what it meant for my prognosis.

Once the post-op nurse determined that I was awake and in good enough shape to go to a room, a hospital transport staff member rolled me away with John trailing after us. I was taken to "John's ward" and into a largish corner room on the third floor of the hospital. The floor nurse, Laura, who had worked with John and his patients extensively, got me tucked in and settled. I actually felt pretty good and so relieved to be through the surgery I had dreaded.

John sat with me. I knew it must be bad if John was taking this much time away from work on a Tuesday. Tuesday is his clinic day, and I can barely get him on the phone even if a disaster happens to strike. (I schedule my disasters for other days of the week, if possible.) For now, *my* cancer was more important than *other people's* cancer. John started calling people—my parents, his parents, my sister—to let them know I had come through the surgery fine, but that they had found cancer in the lymph nodes, and that was all we knew for now. After a while, he left to go home and take care of the kids while I dozed and ate some dinner.

Despite what I was in the hospital for, taking a break from the world is not a bad thing. No phone calls, no e-mails, no expectations. I actually got some sleep, and my mood was fairly good. There were lots of warm blankets and kind staff who seemed to care only about my needs despite, I knew, having to care for quite a few other patients, many in much worse shape than I was. There were cancer patients who were now sick enough to be in the hospital, either because of their cancer or because of their chemotherapy side effects. John knew all the staff, and they knew him, but it also meant that some of his patients were on that floor. However, he managed to excuse himself from encounters with his patients or their family members with a quick, "My wife just had surgery. She's down the hall. I need to run." I was already headline news in the John Marshall fan club.

In the hospital, of course, people constantly go in and out of your room to take blood pressure, change an IV bag, bring food, and clear away food. Each visit meant being roused from sleep. At about 11:30 at night, the new shift of nurses and aides got oriented to the patients, and this time I couldn't go back to sleep. I turned on the television, which is often my sleeping pill. David Letterman was on, and his guest was George Clooney. I happen to love George Clooney and think he might be the best-looking man in the world (other than John, of course). Somehow with the weird magical thinking and reliance on superstition that one develops when nothing seems to be under your control, I felt as if everything would be all right. George Clooney had appeared as my patron saint on a night when I needed a companion and some reassurance, with his twinkly warm eyes and his intelligent and self-deprecating humor. And I went to sleep.

The next morning, a parade of medical students, residents, and fellows arrived, starting about four o'clock. Each asked the same questions, and each wanted to look at my wound. I know people find this trying in training hospitals, but I delighted in it. I had married John before medical school, had turned pages for him while he studied his cadaver, and had transcribed lectures for the class note-taking service. I had heard his stories of women who are paid to receive one vaginal exam after another to help medical students learn how to perform this important task, and I greatly admired them and their fortitude in the service of medical training. Many understanding patients had contributed immeasurably to John's learning how to be a good doctor and oncologist, and my strong belief in contributing to the common good made me happy for these doctors in training to learn on me. I still didn't have pain, thanks to the anesthesiologist and his nerve blocks, which made it easier to be welcoming and receptive to their questions.

One thing I did not do with them was actually look at the wound. I just wasn't ready. Dr. Willey came in later in the morning to see how I was doing, and she suggested I look at it with her. "I think it just looks like when you were a little girl," she said with a smile. It wasn't that bad. My lack of admiration of my breasts was standing me in good stead. I examined it curiously. The right side of my chest was completely flat. I was fortunate that Dr. Willey is such an experienced and talented surgeon, as my wound was a beautifully straight line across the middle of where my right breast had been. I learned later that many women aren't so lucky. One nurse told me that she had seen a scar that looked like a poodle! The wound went straight across and under my right arm, where they had removed the lymph nodes and where two tubes now emerged from my side. That did look a little bizarre.

After two nights in the hospital, I gingerly put on my new surgical bra, and the nurse helped me put the drains in the pockets, which then attached with Velcro to the inside of the cotton corset. John assisted with my oversized Oxford shirt and the sweatpants I had worn into the hospital. As an aide wheeled me downstairs, I thanked everyone profusely for their excellent care.

I was pretty chatty on the drive home. I had gotten through the surgery alive and so far without incident! It was lovely to be outside again. I wasn't enthusiastic about dealing with my wound and dressings and drains, but I knew that my caregiver wouldn't be queasy and had looked at thousands of wounds over the years. He would know if anything was amiss, and probably more important, assure me that nothing was.

The kids arrived home after school, and I joined in their afternoon activities because that sounded like more fun than sitting at home. I wanted to be with other people. We attended a violin lesson for Emma and a medical appointment for Charlie, and I wondered if people could tell I'd had a breast removed. One advantage of the oversized shirt was that, while I looked like the Michelin man because of the surgical bra and drains under the shirt, my underlying physiology wasn't apparent from the outside. Most of the people we were dealing with knew I had had surgery anyway, so I wasn't trying to hide anything.

After dinner, John and I went upstairs to empty the drains and get me ready for bed. He helped me remove my clothes and put on a new pair of pajamas that buttoned in the front. We left the surgical bra on to hold the drains and to put enough pressure on the wound to prevent bleeding and to facilitate healing. I wondered if this was what women who bound their breasts felt like. John emptied the drains while I squeaked, "Don't pull on them!" I could feel every little tug on the stitch that attached the tube to the skin where it entered my body, but mostly I was apprehensive about this bizarre set-up and its seeming instability. He carefully noted the volume of each drain for "Day 1 evening" on the table we had been sent home with. I brushed my teeth and washed my face awkwardly and incompletely with my left hand and took a bit of Percocet to get through the night. I had had no pain during the day, but Dr. Willey had advised me to "stay ahead of the pain."

I was permitted to shower the following morning for the first time since surgery, which felt delightful. However, it meant unwrapping the dressing and really looking at the stitches threaded in a straight line across where my right breast had been. John got in the shower and helped me clean up and wash my hair. Then he dried me and redressed the wound. We went through the drain routine again and reattached them to my surgical bra before getting me into clothes for the day. He fed us all and then headed off to work after taking the kids to school while I lazed on the sofa.

This routine was repeated for about ten days, and I gradually became more comfortable with emptying the drains and caring for the wound. Having a medical professional in the house when you have a medical problem is a blessing. He could answer most of my questions and concerns. Did the wounds look healthy? Was the drainage in the bulbs normal? No need to call the resident on call or even to worry much about anything.

In terms of my health, the week was uneventful, but socially it was jampacked. One friend showed up with several oversized shirts that buttoned up the front because her mother had had breast cancer, and she knew that I couldn't put things over my head. My sister-in-law sent me a pair of cozy button-up pajamas. Another friend brought the kids home from school almost every day. The husband of a former patient of John's who had died way too early, leaving the husband with young triplets, was a caterer, and he showed up with trays of appetizers that we could cook quickly in the oven to serve the many people he knew from experience would be stopping by to visit. Not having to figure out, shop for, and prepare meals was a huge help, and the love and support one feels through the medium of food is potent.

Not only did I feel the love of our friends, but also my diagnosis seemed to start a gentle shift in my relationship with my husband. In the past, whenever I had a medical problem, John would joke, "You're fine. *My* patients have a *real* disease." I guess my revenge was to go out and *get* a real disease. Whether it was seeing me deal with a life-threatening disease, John's specialty, or whether it was his fear of what that meant for him, I saw changes in his attitude toward me. From the time John started carrying a pager when he was a resident, if I needed to get in touch with him, I paged him. That worked for a while, but eventually he got lax about responding. Once we had children, his response time didn't change. So when I needed an immediate answer on something, we developed a code: If the callback number I entered had a 9 at the end, that meant I needed an answer soon; if it had 99 at the end, it was an emergency. We began to differ over what a 9 meant. I frequently needed an answer on something quickly. "I'm at the grocery store. Do you need anything?" "Do you know where Charlie's shoes are? We're about to be late for school." John began to complain about my "flexible" use of the 9. Once I got breast cancer, all of that changed. To this day, he rarely fails to return my call or answer his cellphone.

Another little point of contention in our marriage was kissing me at his work, where people could see us. I don't mean passionate embraces in the hallway—just a quick peck on the lips as we said good-bye if I had been there for something. Early in his career, I think he felt that kissing his wife at work made him look weak or less professional, so he asked that we not do it anymore. I was a bit hurt and thought it was silly, even as I understood why he might feel that way. He was kissing his *wife*, after all. But I complied, although I teased him, "Don't worry, I'm not going to kiss you." All that changed. The hospital had become *my* healthcare venue, and my situation was dire. So kissing me in the hall seemed more like an expression of intimacy and support than imposing our private life on his professional one.

Our marriage had been stable up to my diagnosis. Maybe that is damning with faint praise, but that meant it still existed, and our children didn't have to listen to nightly arguments. I had experienced the constant disdain for my father that my mother had conveyed throughout my lifetime. But John and I had fallen in love passionately in October 1981, and we spent every minute together that we could.

Even after we married, we continued to be each other's lover and best friend as we navigated our developing careers. We found time to be together in any way we could even if it meant my taking John dinner while he was on call or John bringing me lunch as I sifted through documents for discovery in a legal case. We were overjoyed when we found out that I was pregnant with Charlie, and parenting our children was a team activity. However, children have a way of pulling you in different directions, both physically and figuratively, and our jobs did that as well. John saw an increase in his influence concomitant with his work. The resulting increase in the domestic jobs that fell to me fed my desire to have some influence *outside* the house, which led to my taking on more and bigger volunteer activities. So our marriage became predictable: sex once a week, whether we wanted to or not, happy dinners as a family when John was home, and not much time to listen to what the other one really felt or wanted. It wasn't estrangement, but no longer the deeply intimate relationship we had enjoyed. Maybe that's what it was like for everyone. We just didn't imagine that it would be that way for us as well.

I reveled in my week at home with dispensation to do nothing. I snoozed in front of the television in the family room as the family swirled around me. I took things easier than usual in late November with Christmas fast approaching, although I did do a lot of online Christmas shopping. I enjoyed the attention that I received and the frequent reminders that I was surrounded by a warm and supportive community of friends. I particularly enjoyed the attention from John. He left work early and was home in the late afternoon. He monitored and participated in my getting up and going to bed. Even the kids were solicitous of my comfort.

It was an idyllic period, a sort of weird honeymoon time of relief and joy just to have the breast and nodes off me and to have the normal demands on my life reduced. But I knew that this feeling wasn't going to last with the dreaded chemotherapy looming: the attendant hair loss, nausea, pain, and fatigue. And I would have radiation after that. The treatment of my breast cancer wasn't over, not by a long shot.

CHAPTER 7

A Message from Our Sponsor

C ancer always catches people by surprise and will always be someone else's problem, but below the surface, we are all terrified that one day, the someone else will be us.

We live our lives and perhaps experience a few weird symptoms. We go to a doctor, who orders a few *routine* tests and WHAM. Or we are on vacation, (BTW, never go on vacation because that's when everyone gets cancer), typically a cruise, and the dinner buffet doesn't settle well. Our spouse notices that our eyes are a bit yellow, and the ship's doctor freaks out. In Nassau, we are thrown overboard in the nicest possible way. We fly home, go to the local emergency room, get a scan, and WHAM. Then there is a classic. Recently retired and planning how we are going to spend all of that hard-earned money, we get checked by our primary care doctors for the first time in years. They do a test because of some unusual back pain, and WHAM. Or we have had a lot of symptoms, and doctors are ignoring us, and they think it is too much stress when we are sure it is cancer. They advise getting more exercise, and then they notice that we are losing weight and decide to do a scan, and WHAM. Or we are dutifully doing our culturally mandated mammogram, colonoscopy, PSA test, or PAP smear, or having that little spot on our arm checked, knowing that we will be fine. Yes, WHAM.

No one can prepare you for the impact of a cancer diagnosis. Who has the time to deal with doctors, scans, blood tests, and biopsies? We have work, family, trips, lives to live. But a cancer diagnosis immediately puts all such activities on hold. After being told you have cancer, you are too shocked and panicked to hear anything. Thoughts are racing and leading in one unavoidable direction: Is this it? Am I going to die?

There are standard reactions to the WHAM. One is: "Get me in to see anyone at all as fast as you can." The other is: "Who is the best, smartest expert in the world who knows more than anyone ever knew and actually has the cure but is keeping it from the general public but will give it to me because I am so special and well-connected?" We flash to visions of our funeral. We worry that our children will never get into college; they will get married without us. With executive function lost, we are a mess.

Then, remembering the great words of Monty Python that we are "not dead yet," we take charge. We need the best team. Wasn't there an ad on TV this morning about the best cancer center ever? Let's go there! Is the center in our network? In network, out of network, we're not even sure what a network is. We pick up the phone and call. "Welcome to Medstar's Lombardi Cancer Center. If this is a medical emergency, dial 911." We are tempted—this is a fucking emergency after all—but we know better. "Our office hours are 8:00 a.m. until 5:00 p.m. Monday through Friday. Our fax number is slowly being read to you while your mind wanders to the fact that you have cancer. Wait, what was the next option? I think I missed it…. If you are a physician, press 1." (We docs always get 1. We have exclusive access to food in the doctor's lounge, the best parking, the longest white coats, and we walk on water.) "If you are from a hospital or physician's office, press 2." This is business class. "If you know the extension of the party you are calling, press 3." Who on earth knows the extension? "For medical records, hang up and call a totally different number. For doctors A-K, press 4; for doctors G-M, press 5; and for doctors N-Z, press 6. For all other doctors, press 7. If you are a new patient and wish to make an appointment with one of our incredible doctors that you saw on our ad this morning, press 9."

We press 9.

Welcome to the club you never wanted to be a member of. Let's review some basics of the new world you are totally dependent on, your neighborhood cancer center.

Delivering cancer care is complicated. Doing it right requires a well-trained, multi-specialty medical team all aligned in their mission to ease the suffering and sometimes cure a terrible set of diseases. What really makes up a comprehensive cancer center? Operating rooms, operating room staff, lab techs, radiology suites, radiology techs, a CT scanner, a PET scanner, an MRI scanner, radiologists who can read all those pictures, pathologists, microscopes, special stains, genetic testing labs, geneticists, social workers, medical assistants, nurses, nurse practitioners, physician assistants, oncologists, radiation oncologists, pharmacists, robots, cyberknives, proton beam machines, ordinary radiation machines, fiducials (small gold beads—no kidding, gold—inserted into a patient to guide the radiation machines to deliver the radiation to the right spot), gastroenterologists, neurosurgeons, lung surgeons, rehab experts, enterostomal therapists, pulmonologists, dermatologists, lots more "ologists," ICU teams, liver surgeons, pancreas surgeons, peritoneal surgeons, interventional radiologists (these people are really important and are worth double whatever we pay them), palliative care doctors (worth three times what we pay them), nutritionists, art therapists, parking attendants, pagers, page operators, electronic medical records, computers in every room, and many, many more nurses. And if that were not enough, you will get to know a small battalion of administrators who collect your data, interface with insurance companies, and make sure your prescription arrives at the correct branch of CVS.

Hands down the best part of my job is the people with whom I work. Those who seek and accept a job in cancer care are different—in a good way. Our days are filled with emotional-laden challenges coming at us from every direction. Compared with other kinds of medicine, a high percentage of our patients die on our watch. Our day-to-day demands are stressful, resulting in the highest level of burnout throughout our industry. (My competitive nature will celebrate being number one in nearly anything, even this.) At any social function when we are introduced as "oncologists," quickly translated to "cancer doctors," the response is nearly always, "That must be so hard."

When a patient is cured, all the extra effort, the emotion spent, the late nights doing patient notes, and the early mornings keeping up on the latest literature are all justified. We literally high-five each other as we pass in the hall, celebrating our teamwork and skill. It's our version of the touchdown end zone dance, but nerdier. Cured patients give us energy, recharge our batteries, fulfill our purpose, and restore our souls. This is necessary as our batteries are constantly being drained by the many patients who cannot be cured. We have *failed* to cure them. In these cases, the flow of emotional energy is reversed. The patient and family need *our* energy and support. They test our skills, endurance, and compassion. Patients with fatal cancers force us to question the existence of a righteous God, make us lose sleep, and lead us to contemplate a professional question such as whether dermatology would have been a better career choice. Sometimes we go to bed dreading the next clinic day.

I love all my patients, but I love those with metastatic, incurable cancer more. It is these people who really test a cancer center team. How do we deliver what is needed at the worst of times? These people and their bravery, brightness of spirit, and carpe diem priorities provide us with daily reminders of what is really important in life. While our inability to cure them hurts and drains our batteries, it is the care that we deliver at the lowest moments that has the greatest impact. This care can be delivered only with humility and a quiet voice. The best cancer care is delivered when no one else is watching.

Cancer care teams are completely co-dependent, unable to deliver even the most basic cancer care without each other. Cancer patients and families encounter many people during the battle, and we often forget that each one of us has an impact. Virtually every word we say to a patient is valued, craved, and absorbed, all contributing to the total cancer experience. If any member of our team, from the parking attendant to the senior attending physician, says something in the wrong way, fails to do their job perfectly, or does not display the correct level of emotion or compassion, we cause more suffering. Worse, we could get a bad score on Yelp. There is a reason that many centers employ Disney as a consultant: We want everyone to have a magical day.

Cancer is a highly profitable big business, and like all businesses, we advertise. If you are unlucky enough to be awake at 6:47 a.m. and tuned into the morning news shows, I will be there, dressed in my white coat, looking earnest as our team pretends to talk about a tough case. I've been on the side of a bus staring back at morning commuters. I've been on the radio and re-tweeted. I make sure that all our friends and family see the ads, proud to get the shout-outs. We work so hard our claims must be true, right? Our intent is to convince you that we provide by far the best cancer care, and you will die if you go anywhere else.

I cringe, knowing how misleading these ads are, thinking of all the patients who buy into them. The worst are from a national chain of cancer centers. They present an image of exclusivity and greatness, when in fact their business model is designed to milk the most money out of every patient's insurance—they only take patients with private insurance. Their focus on hugs at the door, laughter therapy, and almost fraudulent claims on the impact of nutrition as complements to traditional cancer care are certainly distinguishing in the marketplace but do not result in improved outcomes. They really do make patients feel loved, and their docs and staff are terrific, but their ads prey on the vulnerable, claiming standard-of-care technology as a new discovery that only they provide.

One-stop shopping for cancer care is a better way to go. Cancer patients get a lot of tests and see a lot of doctors. Delivering cancer care in a large, collaborative team is not only easier but also provides better care when we're working together. We can see each other's notes, scans, and labs, enabling a quicker and deeper understanding of a patient's medical story. Over time, we doctors get to know each other, our practice styles, and what we each can and, often more important, cannot do. We run into each other in the doctors' lounge, and we talk about our patients in the hall. We coordinate their care and don't just *say* we will.

In contrast, if someone is having surgery in one system, thinking it has the greatest surgeon in the history of humankind (according to your neighbor's pastor), getting scans at the radiology center at work because it is convenient, and seeing an oncologist in the hospital near the house because it has the best parking lot, then healthcare inevitably will be fragmented and not nearly as good.

A peek inside a cancer center tumor board will show how we typically come to our recommendations. Tumor boards are probably not what you think they are. Each week at Georgetown/Lombardi, more than ten tumor boards meet to review complicated cancer cases. These are multi-disciplinary, attended by surgeons, radiation therapists, oncologists, pathologists, radiologists, social workers, and geneticists. Our students and trainees also are there, mostly to learn through listening in on the discussion. As cancer care is a team sport, tumor boards are the locker room. And as is typical of locker rooms, the press and interestingly the patient who is being discussed aren't included. Sometimes the plan is pretty straightforward. You have a standard problem; we have a standard play to call. Surgery first (pull the weed); oncology second (treat the yard); radiation third (fry the original spot, leaving no roots behind).

But increasingly, cancer cases are complex and require much more than a cut-out standard protocol. The team will need to call a trick play, a flea flicker, individualized for you. Maybe the current science is controversial. Maybe the patient has some social issue—underinsured, no one to help at home, has to keep a job, and the list goes on—which prevents the standard plan from being feasible. Maybe the surgeon who really should do the operation cannot get the patient scheduled for a couple of weeks. Will that delay give the cancer more opportunities to spread? Some countries have laws that require every newly diagnosed case of cancer to be presented at a tumor board. In the United States, where few standards exist across our industry, we can do whatever we want. Live free or die.

For many cases, we know what to do before we meet, but we still want to validate our plan. However, we often present cases in tumor boards when we're not quite sure what to do. We can argue, cite literature, recount our personal experiences, and include our interpretation of the patient's goals and expectations. The decisions often depend on who is in the room, and who has the loudest or the most reasonable voice. We learn from each other, and we teach each other. The result? Patients get better care. Tumor boards are not a formal, algorithmic process. They are a collection of trained but fallible humans trying to help other humans, with all the miracles of human inspiration and human error.

I received a special invitation to the breast tumor board the evening Liza's case was to be presented. I immediately declined. First, my presence would have inhibited free speech. Second, I did not want to know.

Every morning when I walk into work, surveying the shop to make sure the place is still standing, I see our patients waiting in our lobby for us to "open." They have to be there. They don't want to be there. They have no idea what today holds. They have brought breakfast, a newspaper, and their phones to pass the anxious minutes, sometimes hours.

After Liza's diagnosis, I really started to *see* these people. There are a lot of couples. Many are without hair, and some are actually laughing—how can someone on chemo laugh? An older woman has a twenty-year-old granddaughter in tow, maybe the driver, maybe just along to take notes, both doing a jigsaw puzzle in the corner. A man no older than forty sits in a wheelchair, frail, sick, clearly dying, and apparently alone. Patients battling cancer alone are one of our biggest challenges.

Not everyone has a village, but most have at least someone, a friend, a collection of friends. I have no idea how truly single people do it. I spot a couple who resemble Liza and me, and maybe I recognize them. They look normal, well dressed, probably headed to work later, now silently checking their phones. Which one has cancer? It's hard to tell. Both clearly are nervous and appear used to waiting in a familiar place.

I never really noticed them before I became one of them. I never sensed the anxiety or appreciated how much I hated feeling that way, as they surely must. Patients experience the loss of control and the inability to plan because who knows what awaits us. Nothing prepared us for this diagnosis, so there is nothing we can ever prepare for again. Will we be relieved after this appointment or distraught? Will we be planning our next vacation or maybe our bucket list? I cannot stand the feeling of not knowing our future. I need to act, but there the only action is waiting. We all sit and wait, outwardly calm, inwardly a mess.

Since Liza's cancer, I get to work even earlier. I want to make it through the lobby before the couples have arrived, avoiding wading through their tension and uncertainty, avoiding eavesdropping on the voices in their heads. I imagine how their minds have drifted off, perhaps to visions of funerals. The medical assistant calls a name so loudly that you jump. So much for HIPAA privacy rules. You snap out of your daze, gather yourself, and head back. Blood pressure taken, it is higher than ever recorded—we are used to this around here, and we ignore it. The exam room door is closed. You are on the exam table, paper crinkling under you as you shift uncomfortably. Big breaths, flipping through your notes and list of questions, unable to focus on the words. Listening through the door to the conversation next door. You hear laughter again; what kind of place is this?

You hear a stressed conversation in the hall. You hear a light tap on the door, it opens, and in we come.

But not this time. This time I am sitting in that cold room with Liza. And I am not the one knocking on the door; I am on the inside. I am the one dreading what we may hear next.

CHAPTER 8

The In-Between Time

About a week after my surgery, John and I returned to Georgetown to see Dr. Willey for my follow-up visit, where we would learn what the pathologist had found, which would give us some idea about my prognosis. The Breast Center waiting room had become a place of very unhappy associations from my first core needle biopsy when I had the lump in April to my pre-surgery visit, when I was physically chilled by the anxiety of what was to come. The room was associated with so much worry that I was almost shaking every time I walked in there. It wasn't just expecting bad news; it was the *apprehension* about what degree of bad the news would be.

Dr. Willey checked my wound and proclaimed it to be healing nicely. As John sat nearby, she checked the drains and noted the fluid output on John's carefully maintained log sheet, and she decided to remove them. It was an odd feeling as the stitch that held each one in me was snipped and pulled out, the tube slithering along under my skin until the end emerged from my body. Dr. Willey bandaged the small hole that remained, then delivered the news: The pathologist had found that three of the thirteen axillary lymph nodes contained cancer cells, as did three of the six within the breast itself, part of what was known as the "axillary tail." The amount of cancer in each node was "small," Dr. Willey noted encouragingly, and there was "very little invasive disease in the breast." My tumor again tested negative for estrogen, progesterone, and HER-2, so I definitively had triple-negative breast cancer.

The pathology report was more frightening, and the all-caps seemed to emphasize how dramatic it all was. The report began by announcing "DIAGNOSIS: RIGHT BREAST MODIFIED RADICAL MASTECTOMY." The grim news was that I had a "[h]igh grade micropapillary ductal carcinoma demonstrating extensive lymphatic permeating with tumor emboli 2.5 cm in dimension." It also gave me a new piece of information that I had to look up to understand: an Elston score of 8. According to what I could find on the Internet, this score is derived by giving each of three components of the tumor a score of 1 to 3 and adding them all together; the higher the score, the worse the prognosis.[1] Eight out of nine sounded like a great quiz score but a terrible Elston score. The pathology on the lymph nodes from my armpit showed that the first two "demonstrate[ed] metastatic ductal carcinoma" as well, although there was only a small amount in the second node.

In other words, I had Stage 3A breast cancer.

In a kind but clinical way, Dr. Willey delivered the information from the report more succinctly but less technically. John sat next to the exam table, taking it in, asking a few pathology questions I didn't really understand.

Only later did I learn that everyone *really* thought I was going to die. It was an aggressive type of breast cancer, it had moved at lightning

---

1 "Staging and Grade—Breast Pathology," www.pathology.jhu.edu/breast/staging-grade, September 10, 2019.

speed into my lymph system in its search for other places to invade in my body, and the tumor itself appeared lethal under the microscope. Dr. Willey, however, had done this hundreds of times, and she did not let on that my chances of survival were slim. It didn't really matter at this point anyway. We were going forward with treatment no matter what, and I didn't need her to tell me how bad it was.

I *was* more able to cope with the news this time. I knew worse was to come, but at least I had all the information. As always, bad as it was, it could have been much worse: more lymph nodes affected and visible cancer in other parts of my body.

We left Dr. Willey's office and went upstairs to see Dr. Liu, this time as an official patient of the Lombardi Cancer Center. The Lombardi waiting room does its best to be a pleasant and soothing place. I was met with the dulcet sounds of a dulcimer and the murmur of several people sitting at a craft table. I quickly became aware of how different a medical oncology waiting room is from that in a regular doctor's office. Almost everybody is there with at least one other person. A twenty-five-year-old daughter sat with her parents, the mother clearly the one with cancer. Two women who looked to be in their thirties accompanied a third who I assumed to be their mother, solicitously following her into the exam room. There were husbands with wives and wives with husbands.

I was struck by how little anxiety was apparent. Everyone worked very hard to maintain the aura of control, comprehension, and calm. Daughters who probably squabble with their mothers were gentle, smiling, and supportive. So maybe John and I portrayed calm control over our situation. Of course, we knew everyone who worked there, so I was trying to keep it together, trying to look fine, trying to ensure that no one here need be worried or sad because it's all going to be OK.

I sat and completed the paperwork for new patients, had my vitals taken, and was escorted into an examination room. After a few minutes, Dr. Liu appeared. She gave me a quick look of professional sympathy and briskly moved on to inquiring how I was recovering from the surgery. She examined my incision and my drain sites, palpating the area gently with her delicate hands. After the exam, our visit centered around what chemotherapy I was going to have.

The three drugs given to almost everyone with my cancer were Adriamycin, Cytoxan, and either Taxotere or Taxol, two versions of essentially the same drug. That was the standard-of-care treatment. Dr. Liu went over the various ways these drugs could be administered: One way was Adriamycin, Cytoxan, and Taxotere being given together every three weeks for six cycles; a second was "dose dense," which would be first the Adriamycin and Cytoxan every two weeks for four cycles and then Taxol every two weeks for four cycles. Some side effects of the medications would be the inevitable hair loss, which would occur in two to four weeks after beginning the treatment, nausea and vomiting, muscle aches, fatigue, early menopause, damage to the heart, and neurotoxicity. There were a lot of really bad ones, too, such as permanent organ damage and death. I then would need thirty-five sessions of radiation.

We discussed a clinical trial that I might enter, run by the Southwest Oncology Group (SWOG), which conducts a host of different clinical trials. There were four "arms" or possible treatment regimens. One was "dose dense," which would be Adriamycin and Cytoxan every two weeks but for six cycles and then Taxol every two weeks for six cycles. The second arm differed from the first only in that it used twelve weekly doses of Taxol. The third arm was IV Adriamycin with Cytoxan pills for fifteen weeks and then IV Taxol weekly for twelve weeks. The last arm differed from the third only in that the Taxol would be given for just six weeks. A lottery would determine which arm I would be on. Dr. Liu went over another possible trial, which played with a variety of dosing schedules of the main three drugs, but in one arm it added a drug called Gemcitabine, which could lead to more severe side effects. Last, Dr. Liu mentioned a trial of bone drugs known as bisphosphonates such as Fosamax and Boniva, which I could try after I was done with chemotherapy. This was theorized to help prevent metastases to the bone.

Such a daunting load of information and choices in an area I knew absolutely nothing about. I had heard vaguely of these drugs, more on the news than in a clinical setting. I knew that Taxol had been discovered relatively recently and that it came from the bark of the yew tree. All I knew about Adriamycin was that it had a name similar to a wine, Adria, so someone had given John a bottle once as a joke, and it now sat in his office. I knew enough Latin to know that Cytoxan meant something about killing cells. Not that I thought we weren't trying to kill cells, but when you name your drug "cell killer," it sounds likely to cause extensive collateral damage. Because of the intensity of the drugs and regimens we were discussing, I would require an injection the day after each chemotherapy treatment to stimulate the growth of white blood cells to compensate for the fact that the treatment was going to kill a lot of them, leaving me vulnerable to serious infections.

I don't really remember any of this discussion, but throughout it John sat, took notes, and asked many important questions. It is beyond me how couples do this when neither one of them knows anything about cancer treatment or lacks a doctor friend or family member who can untangle the mass of information. Once more, I sat dazed and confused, looking back and forth from John to Dr. Liu, hoping someone would tell me what to do. Dr. Liu told me it was my choice, but I didn't have to make it today. She subtly made it clear though that I was at high risk for metastasis.

Finally, because my grandmother had had breast cancer and because I had an invasive breast cancer before menopause, Dr. Liu recommended that I have genetic testing to see if I carried the BRCA-1 or BRCA-2 gene. Triple-negative breast cancer is the type that people with those genes get. More testing, more big implications.

Dr. Liu's note from that day concluded: "The patient expressed a complete understanding of the information summarized above." I'm sure I did say I understood what she had said. What else could I say? We could have talked for several days, and I still wouldn't have had a complete understanding. But she was required to ask me and document my answer, and I was required in a sense to say I understood.

John always recommends that people with a cancer diagnosis get a second opinion, so he had been looking around for another breast oncologist I might see. There are lots of oncologists in the Washington, D.C., area, many of them excellent, although many are private physicians as opposed to academic physicians, which would mean a different kind of care. Many private doctors have fancy offices with state-of-the-art chairs for chemotherapy infusions in private rooms, each with a television, snacks, and other amenities. There aren't generally fellows and residents who assist in your care, which could be viewed as either positive or negative. The primary mission of a community oncologist is to deliver "standard-of-care" cancer treatment, although many do participate in some clinical research.

On the other hand, an academic oncologist is part of a group whose primary mission is research, so there is access to many trials of either new medicines or different ways of administering older medicines that the researchers believe may be more effective. Many people who start with a private oncologist end up in an academic or research institution for their care because their situation has worsened, and the community oncologist no longer has anything to offer them. The patients are looking for new treatments that might be the "magic bullet" or even just give them a few more months. In addition, in a teaching hospital, one frequently is seen by an oncology fellow before seeing one's treating physician, and residents and fellows are the first line of defense should there be an urgent problem during the off hours.

John admired and respected a doctor who worked at Inova Fairfax Hospital in Virginia and specialized in breast cancer, so he called her to ask if she would see us to discuss options and possible treatment. We went to see her the day after I saw Dr. Liu. Her office was completely different. The office was in a medical office building, not in the hospital, and the waiting room was small and relatively empty. The treatment area was spick-and-span and new. Georgetown University Hospital is not spick-and-span or new. Founded in 1898, it is one of the oldest teaching hospitals in the Washington, D.C., area.[2] It is also constrained by its location in the city in the middle of Georgetown, so it rarely puts up a new building, meaning the administration is trying constantly to keep several older buildings up-to-date. And don't get me started on the parking!

We talked with the Fairfax doctor about my situation, and she gave me a piece of good news I hadn't heard before. She said that although triple-negative has poor outcomes and is likely to recur in 40 to 50 percent of cases, it is most likely to do that in the first three years after surgery. If it doesn't recur then, I could consider myself relatively home free. Many women with other forms of breast cancer, particularly

---

2 "Medstar Georgetown University Hospital," Wikipedia, September 11, 2019.

those with estrogen-positive breast cancer, can have a recurrence even twenty years after diagnosis.[3] It *was* a silver lining in all the gloom and doom I was facing.

She went over the SWOG trial again since her group was participating in it, and she was enthusiastic about it, although she cautioned that one of the arms could "get pretty tiresome." She also offered another trial that used the drug bevacizumab, commonly known as Avastin, which would be given after the Adriamycin/Cytoxan cycles.

I was torn. I liked her. I liked her office although it seemed a bit sterile. I like old buildings and was used to Georgetown's charm and personality. I could get on the SWOG study with her as well, which I was leaning toward. It would be really inconvenient for John, though, as her office was in the opposite direction from Georgetown. Also, I couldn't drive myself there or home because of the drugs I would be given to help me tolerate the chemotherapy. I certainly wasn't unaware or unappreciative of the strong advantages to being at a place where everyone knew me.

After thinking it over, I let Dr. Liu know that I wanted to be treated at Georgetown and that I wanted to enroll in the SWOG study. John seemed to be in favor of it, I assumed both because he wanted me to do a clinical trial and because he thought more chemotherapy was likely to be better. For me, it sounded as if it would have the most benefit with the least likely detriment. As I said before, I just wanted to spray Raid down my throat to get rid of the cancer cells that were still in me, so more chemotherapy than the standard of care sounded like the next closest and probably safest thing.

---

3 "Breast Cancer Recurrence Risk Lingers Years after Treatment Ends," labblog. uofmhealth.org/body-work, September 11, 2019.

John seemed oddly removed from the decision-making process. He hadn't really told me anything about my situation, about the poor prognosis of triple-negative breast cancers. He was willing to answer my questions, which he did calmly and carefully, but he didn't want to escalate my anxiety by volunteering all he knew. His reluctance to discuss also might have been for his own protection. Reminding himself of the likelihood that I wasn't going to make it, preceded most likely by months if not several years of debilitating treatments, was not useful for his own state of mind. He knew that I don't take bad news well from him and realized that if he did pass on unpleasant and unwelcome facts, he might suffer some of the consequences. Occasionally he would come home from some event in the next few years and try to encourage me by telling me brightly that he had met someone whose wife had had triple-negative breast cancer, and she was still alive over five years later! I found gleaning some reassurance from this difficult. Instead, I thought, "Great, if 50 to 60 percent of women with this disease survive, then there's someone who's taken one of those spots, so fewer are left for me."

This was the second clinical trial I had enrolled in, the first being the one that yielded my diagnosis. I am a big believer in clinical trials, and John resembled an evangelical minister about them. In *The Emperor of All Maladies,* Pulitzer-winning author Siddhartha Mukherjee observes that the progress of cancer treatment has been quite slow, and the treatments continue to be rather barbaric (as I was soon to experience). One reason for this, as John would continually preach, was that only about 3 percent of all cancer patients enroll in clinical trials, although parents of children with cancer had enrolled their children at a rate of 98 percent over the years. As a result, advances in the treatment of pediatric cancers have been far more rapid than those for the treatment of adult cancers. Even without John's indoctrination, my own community-oriented tendencies meant that I was not only eager to participate in clinical trials but also felt a responsibility to do my part in advancing the treatment of breast and other cancers. In the end, I was really scared and willing to do anything, suffer anything, put up with anything to make the cancer go away.

So off to the SWOG trial I went.

When you're doing things to people that are designed to cure them but might kill them, you have to take a lot of precautions. Before I started taking (or, more accurately, being given) Adriamycin, which can cause congestive heart failure down the road, I needed to have a MUGA (multiple-gated acquisition) scan. This scan would look at the lower chambers of my heart to check whether they were pumping blood properly and would give a baseline for future scans.

So a few days after meeting with Dr. Liu, I returned to nuclear medicine, my new favorite department, where a tech took some of my blood and mixed it with some radioactive material as a tracer. He sent me off to wait for the blood and radioactive material to mingle properly before he injected my blood back into a vein. Then yet another large, noisy machine whirred around my unmoving body for an hour. Fortunately, my heart was in good shape. The more I learn about cancer treatment, the more I realize how lucky I was to be in generally good health because this freed the doctors to go in "guns blazing." Not everyone is so lucky, which means that medical oncologists, surgeons, and radiation oncologists have to alter treatment to work around patients' other medical issues.

When I look back at my calendar from the day of the MUGA, December 6, 2006, I am amazed at all we managed to pull off during that period. On that day alone, we dropped Charlie off at 7:45 a.m.

at a high school to which he was applying, and we met him there at 11:00 a.m. for a family interview. I had the heart test at 1:00 p.m. at Georgetown, and our meeting with the oncologist I was considering was at 3:30 p.m. Somehow Charlie made it to the dentist at 3:30 to follow up on his braces, Emma took a piano lesson at 6:00 p.m., and Charlie got to Boy Scouts at 7:00 p.m. One assumes that we all ate dinner, but maybe that was more than we could handle. My calendar seems to indicate that we incorporated the new medical demands into our normal lives. I suppose we did, but only with massive amounts of help from my parents and the friends we soon would rely on even more.

CHAPTER 9

The Standard of Care Is Unacceptable

The standard of care for Liza's cancer was to give "AC followed by T." The breast cancer research machine had figured out that compressing higher doses closer together, called "dose dense," cured more patients than when the doses were lower and more spread out. This wisdom was the result of a series of large trials designed to find small improvements. Sure, dose dense was more toxic, but so worth it! However, with little mature data specific to triple-negative breast cancer, this total treatment package was thought to increase Liza's odds of being cured by about 20 percent or so, from not very good to a little better.

We were interested in better odds than that. Behind curtain number two was "the trial," a national study being done by what we call a cooperative group. Cooperative groups are not well named. There are several of them, teams of cancer centers that agree to work together to do clinical research. This is the cooperative part. But all these centers are highly competitive because they are composed of scientists and clinical researchers who are competing for the lead, for academic recognition. Think college sports conferences, ACC, SEC, Big 10. On one level you compete, but on another you need each other, and you share a common identity. Sure, we Dukies hate the Tar Heels, but we are both allied to hate Kentucky even more.

The groups are funded at least partially by the National Institutes of Health. Drug companies also help fund some studies, but we recognize that when funded by large drug companies, the objective interests of trials can be lost. Cooperative groups are to be the keepers of truth, refining therapies without a financial interest, focusing only on the patient's best interest. Studies that come out of the cooperative groups are among the "cleanest," uninfluenced by industry motives.

After Liza's mastectomy, we met with Minetta in an examination room to hear about her treatment options. The trial Minetta offered her involved being randomized to one of four different "arms" or treatment plans. In all four arms, AC was followed by T; the same basic drugs but on different schedules. All four arms were some modification of the standard treatment, trying to answer the question of whether longer treatment was better than shorter, and if the schedule of administration of every week versus every two weeks matters. Whichever arm she was randomized to, Liza would get a research arm. Her fate was in the hands of the randomization gods.

Claudine joined us, and we immediately lapsed into oncologist shorthand. I impatiently asked questions about the mechanics and schedules of each treatment arm, and Claudine and Minetta shot back learned answers. I looked at Liza as we discussed all these options, and she looked at all of us with a bewildered expression on her face. I know she was grateful (I think I know she was grateful), but I also know this couldn't have been easy. We were deciding her fate. We gave her the illusion of having a choice, but in the end, all the arrows pointed in one direction: We were in.

For someone whose life is clinical research, I reacted oddly. Despite all my questions in the office, I never asked about the design of the trial. I never read the background information on why the SWOG cooperative breast sub-committee felt that this was such a good trial. Why these specific arms? What justification was there for extending the treatment longer than standard? I never looked into the statistics to find out how big the trial was, nor did I ask what delta they were looking for. I am an expert at reading trials, and I review them each month for our cancer center to assess the quality of the science. It would have taken me all of five minutes to review the trial.

But I didn't.

I didn't even read her consent form, the document meant to describe in detail the added risk. I never asked the most important question: What was the chance the treatment was going to kill her? I knew it was low, but I also knew it was not zero. As a final reassurance of any big decision in my clinic, my patients regularly ask if our agreed-upon plan is what I would do for my wife or for my father. I never asked Claudine or Minetta the age-old question, "If Liza were your sister, what would you do?"

I still wonder why. I told myself that I needed to be the caregiver, not her doctor. I had overseen the building of the system that would treat Liza. I needed to trust it; somehow, I felt I had to trust it *blindly*. If I questioned the treatment recommendations that Liza received, would I not need to question all treatment recommendations any of us made? Plus, my lack of inquisitiveness was an expression of complete trust in our doctors. I knew that for this team, treating Liza was tantamount to treating their best friend or their sister.

As long as I am taking inventory of all my lapses, I must include the fact that I did no research into her specific cancer. I have never read her full path report, having been traumatized by the path report I did see. I haven't looked at her scans. I turned down the invitation to hear her case presented in the tumor board. In the official caregiver handbook, Chapter 1 covers being supportive and always present for your loved one. Chapter 2, right there in black and white, is titled, "DO RESEARCH ABOUT THE DISEASE TO MAKE SURE YOUR LOVED ONE'S CARE IS APPROPRIATE, STATE OF THE ART, AND WE ARE NOT MISSING ANYTHING OUT THERE THAT IS BETTER." I still never have.

Right after her diagnosis, I couldn't. I left any noon lecture that was on triple-negative breast cancer, even if pizza was served. I knew how much trouble she was in; I knew what was ahead for her, from the acute treatment to the painful, anxious waiting game. But I did not question things. Liza's doctors were terrific, and they were my close colleagues. If they thought this was the right thing to do, it was the right thing to do.

The randomization gods assigned Liza to the most aggressive treatment arm, and off we went to press beyond the standard of care. I understood what was likely to happen to Liza, and it was going to be rough.

I had no idea what was about to happen to me.

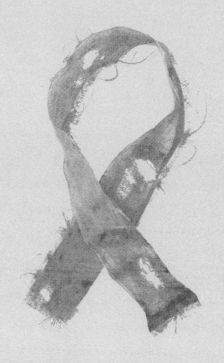

PART 3

Finding Value in Cancer Care

Opening Lecture of the Otto J. Ruesch Center Annual Symposium
Georgetown University
Washington, D.C.
December 2009

ood morning and welcome! I am so pleased to see all of you here at the first of what I hope to be many annual Ruesch Center Symposia, Fighting a Smarter War on Cancer. We hope you will find our content and format different from those of the other meetings you attend. Our goal is lofty. We want to tackle the big issues that we face as a cancer community and in particular what might be slowing our progress in GI cancers. We have invited a terrific faculty to help us define the key concerns, and we have challenged them to propose some solutions.

I would like us to begin by discussing the complex subject of cancer economics, specifically the concept of value in healthcare, a subject that I am obsessed with, and wrote about in a piece for the Washington Post. *Since I am sure most of you didn't read it, let me share some of the key points.*

When President Richard Nixon declared his "war on cancer," healthcare was not the overwhelming economic problem it is today. In 1970, healthcare expenditure was only about 7 percent of the U.S. gross domestic product; today it is nearly 18 percent. By 2020, U.S. healthcare costs are expected to be so high that the country's health-care system would, on its own, comprise the fourth-largest economy in the world, and nearly 10 percent of this total is being spent on cancer care. As we have made dramatic progress on tackling infectious diseases globally, cancer is quickly becoming the number one public health issue for all nations.

When I began my career, cancer research involved an intimate collaboration among all the major stakeholders. Representatives from government, industry, and academics were all welcome to the same table. The best minds working together and in competition, as is common in the research world, were modestly supported by our taxes through the National Cancer Institute budget and a growing investment from the pharmaceutical industry. As an academic researcher with an expertise in GI cancers and new drug development, I was honored to be included. We weren't worried about or ever really aware of conflicts of interest and who was paying for what. People were dying of cancer. We were at war. Our cause was urgent—we will figure all that other stuff out later, after the victory.

Even while we made steady progress, the world of cancer research gradually changed, a shift that was felt by those of us in the trenches. A watershed moment was the discovery of paclitaxel, trade name Taxol, a drug that my wife, Liza, would receive fourteen years after its Food and Drug Administration approval. Federally funded researchers at NCI actually discovered paclitaxel at a cost to the U.S. taxpayers of more than $400 million, a terrific investment of our national resources. Since the U.S. government was not in the business of manufacturing drugs, for a bargain-basement price of $35 million, our government sold the rights to the pharmaceutical company BMS, which manufactured and marketed the drug to the tune of a $9 billion revenue stream. Our oncology community recognized the irony of the disproportionate profit from government research, but we needed BMS to help fight our war on cancer—in the same way that we need Lockheed Martin, General Dynamics, and Northrop Grumman for supplies to fight traditional wars. Few people argued that this sweet government contract wasn't worth it in the end. Of course it was.

In just a few years, cancer became "big business." Due to a deliberately placed loophole in our regulatory laws, it is against the law for our government healthcare programs, Medicare in particular, to negotiate the price of healthcare. We are the only country on the planet where this is true. As a result, manufacturers, hospitals, and doctors can charge whatever they wish, and for the most part, they expect to be paid close to the asking price. This system feeds on insurance, as no one really could afford any healthcare without someone else picking up the tab. As you sit here today, would you swipe your own Visa card to pay for a new cancer drug for you or your family? Could you actually afford the enormous sticker prices that provide only modest clinical benefit? Would you be able to make a value decision for your healthcare as we all do when buying virtually anything? Is what I am about to buy worth it? When pressed, most of us would say no, too expensive for the return. In such a world, most cancer care would not meet a traditional value assessment.

The big disconnect that is somehow lost on the American public is that we are all picking up the healthcare tab, just indirectly. Our paychecks are lower, and our taxes are higher, and our national debt grows ever larger all because of the rising cost of healthcare. Nowhere has the rapid rise of healthcare costs been more easily tracked than the price of cancer care and specifically cancer drugs. With every new innovation, every new diagnostic tool, and especially every new drug, prices skyrocketed. Publicly, these escalating prices were explained, even justified, by similarly escalating research and development costs. But those of us in R and D knew better. Our research costs were not changing appreciably, so why were theirs? Their answer? Innovation was expensive, and we should be grateful for the discoveries. Just shut up and pay.

Thus, we enter the roaring nineties of cancer drug development, and what a feeding frenzy it was. Everyone got in the game, which is best *explained in an easy four-step process. Step one: Invent a new cancer therapy. It's not required to be a blockbuster because it needed only to be a little better than the one before. In fact, it could be a "me too" drug copying a competitor's idea. Step two: Perform a large clinical trial showing a small but statistically significant benefit. Step three: After FDA approval, charge a lot more than anyone ever charged before. Step four: Make lots of money off our disconnected, insurance-supported healthcare system. The hospitals and doctors were happy about the escalating costs. Under our current model, we resell the drugs at a markup. The dirty little secret is that doctors are incentivized to prescribe more expensive drugs.*

All of this was in the name of progress in the war on cancer. The insurance companies passed on the costs to the public, not willing to suggest that progress in cancer care, regardless of how small, was somehow not worth it. Was not this the best use of our money?

We all got greedy. We lost our objectivity and our innocence. One of our darkest hours involved the use of "growth factors" to stimulate the bone marrow of cancer patients undergoing chemotherapy treatment. Our cancer drugs were beating up patients' bone marrows, limiting our ability to push doses even higher, not only the fashion of the day, but also a principle we fundamentally believed would result in more cures. The only way to achieve more breakthroughs with traditional chemotherapy was to increase doses, but we were thwarted by side effects on the bone marrow. To counter this, drugs were invented to stimulate both red blood cell and white blood cell production. The drugs did what they were intended to do. By increasing red cells, we prevented anemia, and by increasing white cells, we rescued patients from the side effects of our more intensive doses of chemo. I saw this firsthand when my wife was fighting breast cancer, and she received this therapeutic strategy. All good, right?

And now, the dark side of the story begins.

The manufacturer convinced everyone that having a higher red count was good; patients would feel better, stronger, and less fatigued, and have a better quality of life. While trials never really proved these aims, oncologists fell in love with these drugs. Sure, they were expensive, but we could justify giving them to a high proportion of our patients, and with each dose we gave, we made money. We made so much money that almost overnight, oncologists became the highest-paid subspecialists among all internal medicine subspecialists. We took in more than cardiologists, gastroenterologists, and pulmonologists, the previous record holders.

We built opulent cancer centers with fancy lobbies, huge infusion units with tropical fish tanks, art therapy, piano music, and valet parking—a cross between Saks and the Beverly Hills Hospital. As the years advanced, one treatment center grew more posh than the next. Despite my best efforts, our infusion unit at Georgetown is still the original model. Cramped, tired, and worn, it's more like an old Sears, nothing like Saks. I knew this crazy, warped system was not going to last forever, and if we didn't fix up our center asap, we would miss the gravy train. For the record, I failed. I never won the argument with our management, and believe me, I tried. Our industry and therefore our personal livelihoods became totally dependent on the resale of cancer treatments.

Then things backfired. It wasn't exactly a 1929 crash, more like a crack in the dike that eventually released a disastrous flood. While we were all shooting up our growth factors and humming "We're in the Money," new results of additional clinical trials surfaced regarding the safety of red cell growth factors. In the name of selling even more drugs, the company designed studies to push red cell levels even higher, "blood doping" for cancer patients. Unexpectedly, the results showed that patients on the experimental doses of the red cell growth factor, and as a result with higher red cell levels, died sooner. Drugs that Liza received, that I administered to her, actually might have shortened her chances for survival. This strategy, intended to make cancer fun again, was harming patients. The FDA withdrew approvals of these drugs, removing major sources of revenue for many cancer service lines and pissing everyone off. But here is the crazy part: Even after the use of the red cell growth factors rapidly declined, causing a dip in our enthusiasm, our business model did not change, and it still hasn't.

I was both witness to and participant in all of this. Yes, our center profited, but I could not help but see our focus lost. Our patients thought we were curing them when in fact we were proclaiming "significant," "major," and "huge" progress for small, modest advances, gains that were not equal to the escalating costs. Somehow, with all this money flowing through our system—from the patient's pockets to insurance companies and taxes for Medicare, to our doctors, hospitals, and drug companies— we must be making proportionate progress.

We were not.

What about thinking more rigorously about value: How much does it cost, and how much benefit does it provide? Somehow, we should be fighting a smarter war on cancer.

*I may appear to be another of those crazy guys you see standing in front of the White House, wearing only a sandwich board sign. On one side in big print is: "I HAVE THE ANSWER TO THE HEALTHCARE CRISIS," and on the other: "THE END OF THE WORLD IS COMING." Certainly, my family has put me in that category. But I just can't stop. We **must** embrace value. You see, by fighting a smarter war, progress actually will accelerate, and advances will be larger and more significant. We will get to cures faster. There will be plenty of healthcare to go around if* *only we use our current resources more wisely. We need to get the word out: "PEOPLE, YOU ARE PAYING FOR YOUR HEALTHCARE. STOP CONSUMING IT AS IF IT WERE FREE!"*

And yet, if we applied a value metric to our current treatments, many therapies would not make the cut. Unfortunately, my wife and I had the opportunity to experience all this firsthand. Liza has given me permission to share this story, mainly because it makes me look pretty bad....

In an instant, Liza's diagnosis of extremely aggressive breast cancer flipped my perspective from vilifying our dysfunctional policies of healthcare to wallowing in the unlimited access Liza and I had as individual consumers. No cancer-fighting weapon was out of reach as she and I faced the loaded gun pointed directly at her. We had good insurance. We had caring, attentive doctors and nurses. We had drugs, the best drugs. We had growth factors at the cost of thousands of dollars each. I was gladly injecting them into her arms, knowing that insurance was paying, knowing that we were ringing up a huge tab. With the gun pointed at you, you don't care. Spend whatever it costs today, and we will worry about paying the bill tomorrow.

Maybe I was being too cheap. How could my more restrained use of expensive therapies have any impact on the national healthcare debt? I was only one of thousands of oncologists. Why should I be the cheap one? Who cares how much it costs?

The problem is that we all should. The reason I am so focused on this issue of value is that we are going to price ourselves out of further innovations and new treatments that our GI cancer patients are praying for so desperately. Our speakers today will drill down on many of the issues I have raised. We waste so much. We overtreat so many and expose patients to treatments and side effects that likely add little benefit. We must embrace value in healthcare. By doing so, we will be forced to refocus away from marginal gains and toward approaches with truly significant improvements. We need innovations that we all see as worth it, treatments that we would gladly whip out our Visa cards and swipe for.

CHAPTER 10

Home or Away

When Liza and I make any family decision, we do the research. We check *Consumer Reports*, we read reviews, and we go to stores to get "up close and personal" on all big-ticket items. Sometimes it can take hours to decide on a restaurant—don't want to eat bad food or miss an opportunity to experience something unique. We read all the guidebooks we can find to optimize our vacation experience. We are pretty tedious to be around, frankly. No wild and crazy, no spontaneous for us.

Why should breast cancer treatment be any different from any other major life decision? This was my world, I knew the options, and I knew the players. Liza was familiar with all this if only by osmosis. She knew a lot of the vocabulary, she had a sense of what was ahead, but when it came to the details, she was still a novice. I had always valued second opinions for my patients. In fact, I regularly recommended that if I were the only oncologist they had seen, then they should get a second opinion. This stuff is too serious, too nuanced, too filled with bias to have only one source of information. Liza and I needed to do this, too, even if we were only going through the motions.

We visited one other provider, another good friend who is also a recognized breast expert but did not work at Georgetown. She was in our community, but getting an opinion outside Georgetown seemed more important for me than for Liza. I wanted Liza to feel she could get treatment somewhere that was hers, not mine. I wanted her to feel comfortable with her team, feel that she could ask questions and share complaints as required. If we were treating her, I would consider every shortcoming of our delivery of her care, real or perceived, as personal. As the one in charge of the shop at Georgetown, I was the complaint department. If she needed more separation from me and more privacy than she would get at Georgetown, then I wanted her to have that option.

We found the oncologist's office, located among a maze of medical office buildings, nowhere near her practice's affiliated hospital, with ample free parking. The waiting room was large and classy, with unworn furniture, more chairs than patients, and the inevitable fish tank. We were checked in politely and received efficiently—no one recognized me. We quickly were called back to meet with the doctor and escorted down a hall; there were no signs of nurses, no phones ringing, no hallway conversations among the staff. We were "roomed" in an almost luxurious exam room, with a new exam table, a functioning blood pressure cuff, and clean floors. We couldn't hear anyone else talking through the walls. I was uncomfortable and very jealous.

My friend was fabulous, the model of confident compassion. She was both hopeful and frank about Liza's situation. She offered the same trials that Minetta had offered and described less-intense standard-of-care options. She then showed us around her infusion unit, with private rooms, sliding glass doors, flat-screen TVs, and enough space for the patient and a caregiver or two. Nowhere was the hustle and bustle of our shop—the noise, the tension, the train station atmosphere. Her space was a yoga studio that also gave chemo. We loved the experience. We both could envision Liza getting her care there, which we knew would be wonderful. I tried to voice no opinion, as this was meant to be Liza's choice.

As we walked out, we talked a bit and compared notes. I asked what she wanted to do, but she wasn't ready to decide. I contained myself. I wanted her to pick Georgetown. I wanted her to be close, to receive treatment in a place that I understood and could influence. I wanted our team to give her chemo, read her scans, park her car. I wanted everyone to know that MY WIFE was being treated there. Our team would not only be on their toes but also take amazing care of her. Our breast team is world renowned, a very deep bench. With Minetta on point, I could almost relax and, at least for Liza's care, forget my role as the boss and focus on my role as the husband.

On the other hand, convenience and familiarity could come at a price. Liza does not trust my medical judgment, at least not in my treating our family. She may ask my opinion, but then conclude that my answer is too cavalier, not addressing the issue. "I am going to ask a real doctor" is a sentence I have heard often from her. What if I was actually on call when something happened? Could I ignore her low-grade fever, knowing it is likely nothing but could be the beginnings of fever/neutropenia, a potentially lethal complication? What about late-night vomiting, diarrhea, bleeding, unusual headaches, some new pain? No way could I be objective. I dreaded being put in that position. Maybe we should get our care from the non-Georgetown doctor so I would be off the hook.

We talked about it for a few days, and then Liza chose Georgetown. I was relieved.

After Liza's surgery, she was given a room in the unit I was responsible for. Her nurse was someone I knew quite well, who not only fussed over Liza but also fussed over me. As I walked out of the hospital unit that first night and looked into the other patients' rooms, many of them my patients, I was amazed that even at this late hour, many were accompanied by their caregivers at the bedside, watching TV, reading, sleeping alongside their loved one, doing what caregivers do. It left me wondering if we could provide the caregiver level of care Liza was receiving for all our patients. I looked up and promised that if we got out of this, I would do what I could to provide that for all.

That first evening, I was comforted to know that our staff, in many ways my extended family, was watching over her. Returning the next morning, I saw Liza sitting up, the sun warming the room, and our nursing team giving her the first lessons on the lovely topic of drain management. From the beginning, seeing Liza cared for by our team, in familiar surroundings, made the entire experience easier for me. Despite the catastrophe, I realized how unbelievably lucky I was. I know our team treats all patients like family, but for me, our team *was* my family. They were going to sweat the small stuff, and they were going to be our care team *and* our caregivers. They were going to be *my* caregivers.

CHAPTER 11

Chemo Day 1

About three weeks after surgery, Dr. Willey examined me and concluded that I could begin chemotherapy and physical therapy. I was struck by the fact that even though both end in "therapy," the two could hardly be more different: One is designed to rebuild strength and flexibility, while the other is designed to kill lots of cells. My first "dose" of each was on Monday, December 18. Every two weeks for the next twenty-four weeks, until May 2007, Mondays would be my chemotherapy day. In the dead of winter, May seemed a terribly long way off. But I am a planner, and I could start organizing ways to cover my duties on those alternate Mondays and the ensuing days when I wouldn't feel good. Both Dr. Liu and John described the rhythm of the treatment: I should expect to feel nauseated the first few days after treatment, then side effects would reach their high point, and perforce I would reach my low point about a week afterward. Then I would gradually improve until the next treatment a week later.

But first I went to physical therapy, which was completely delightful. PT was normally done in a large room with lots of other patients, but because mine required my chest to be exposed so the therapist could massage my scar to minimize scar tissue and to rehabilitate my pectoral muscles, we were secluded. She worked on the area under my arm as well, and went over the things that Dr. Willey had listed to avoid on that arm, adding a few: heat and direct sunlight, hot tubs, tight clothing, and anything medical, such as taking blood pressure or having an injection. She told me that I should get a compression sleeve to wear when I fly, I should wear gloves when I garden, and I should wear long sleeves as much as possible.

This didn't sound like any fun at all. No tennis, no golf, no weight-lifting, no sun, no hot tubs. Never mind the things I needed to do, such as gardening, carrying my suitcase on a plane, bringing in the groceries. I knew lymphedema wouldn't be fun either—chronic swelling and pain—but was the prevention going to be worse than the problem? I didn't think that allowing my arm to wither away sounded like a good approach either. I prodded and pushed back on the restrictions, but I failed to get any different answers.

I decided not to worry about it for now. I would visit the therapist regularly, do my exercises religiously, and eventually figure out what I was willing to give up and what I was willing to run the risk of lymphedema over. Therapy itself was a welcome break from everything else. We chatted about movies, exercise, and our weekends while the therapist massaged the area around the incision.

From physical therapy, I made my way up to the infusion unit in Georgetown Hospital. The first person I saw was the unit secretary, whose daughter had babysat for our children. It was nice to see a familiar face and to be so warmly welcomed. I was escorted into a former hospital room with a bed, a reclining chair, and a bathroom.

Soon I met Mercedes Watson, the heart and soul of this unit, which is limited to patients who are on clinical trials. It seemed as if she had worked with clinical research patients forever. Mercedes is the model of an ideal chemotherapy infusion nurse—exceedingly competent, never flustered, funny, loving. She arrived with her palette of needles and tubes to start my IV. My mood quickly shifted, and suddenly I was petrified. As I already have mentioned, I always have hated needles and have to steel myself for shots. IVs were even worse, despite all my recent experience with them.

Dr. Liu had mentioned the option of having a mediport implanted, which would mean many fewer "sticks." A mediport is a device implanted next to the collarbone during a short outpatient surgery performed by an interventional radiologist. With a mediport, a patient's vein can be accessed both to infuse chemotherapy and to take blood for labs through a small port that sits just under the skin, connected by a tube to a large vein. The needle used to access the port is slim, very short, and therefore not painful because it doesn't need to go into a vein or even very far into the body. Numbing cream is put on the spot before the needle is inserted. One of the drugs I was receiving, Adria-mycin, is especially damaging to veins or anything else it touches. Arm veins are small and almost the sole access to blood and for IVs. In my case, my right arm was out of commission. That meant that my left arm veins would have to do all that work for the rest of my life, so saving them from further abuse would seem to make sense. But despite the strong arguments in favor of a mediport, I decided against it. I had just been through major surgery and had dealt with anesthesia, wounds, doctors, and procedures for several weeks. I wasn't up to doing more of it. In retrospect, that probably was not a good choice, but it seemed to make sense at the time.

Despite my trepidation, I managed to keep my arm still, and Mercedes quickly got an IV started. Chemotherapy nurses are understandably among the best at starting IVs. (When I was in labor with Charlie, and the labor and delivery nurse was having trouble starting an IV, John offered to call one of the Lombardi nurses to do it for her!)

The first infusion of each chemotherapy cycle would be of an anti-nausea drug and steroids, the latter to enhance the effect of the former. Then Mercedes returned with "the red devil." Adriamycin, the drug that most strongly argued in favor of a mediport, is called "the red devil" because of its red color and harsh side effects. It can immediately damage tissue it touches, so it frequently is given by a nurse out of a large syringe rather than from an IV bag hung on a pole with the patient unattended. Should there be any signs of the drug leaking out of the vein, the nurse can immediately stop the infusion. Mercedes warned me that my urine would be tinged with red for the next few days as the Adriamycin cleared my system. I wondered what it was doing to my renal system as well.

We sat, and Mercedes tried to distract me, asking about my family (things she never forgot) and myself. But we both sat transfixed by the slow lowering of the plunger of the large syringe, watching the red liquid flow steadily through the tube that entered my arm. It didn't take long, just twenty minutes or so, and I made it through the first administration of the red devil unscathed. The next drug was the Cytoxan. This was given in the traditional way through an IV bag hung on a pole, and it took about an hour and a half. During the five to six hours I was in the infusion unit every other week, I was able to be on my own, watch television, nap, and write Christmas cards.

I didn't intend to take this year off from my annual Christmas card writing, despite my right arm being in a delicate state from the surgery and the rest of me being in a delicate state from chemotherapy. I had decided not to tell people about my cancer in the Christmas cards. When I started writing them around Thanksgiving, I didn't know much, so I didn't want to say anything. Also, telling people you have breast cancer in a Christmas card seems like a big bummer—not the message I wanted to convey. If people needed to know, we would get that information to them in other ways. It was lovely to have the extra time to do something that felt not only normal, but also special and happy.

I didn't even need to worry about the kids too much. I took them to school in the morning, and my parents took over after school. My parents really jumped into the breach in full force. They had always been generous about being on call for us, and they handled everything from morning until evening with the children and the dog on the days I was in chemo.

Yet, for all their generosity and engagement, something else was going on that was difficult for me: They never asked me how I was or even mentioned the reason they were doing all this. The day we got the diagnosis, my parents barely acknowledged it to me and quickly vanished when we arrived at their house to talk to the children. They probably found it too difficult to handle. I know they cared and worried, and perhaps *because* they cared and worried so much, they couldn't say the words. But I was hurt, and the hurt grew with each round of chemotherapy, particularly as my mother-in-law called the day after each cycle to check in on me, bringing my parents' silence into stark relief.

My parents were of the generation born at the beginning of the Depression and in high school during World War II. Certainly that generation had developed a level of stoicism not seen today, but their lack of emotional engagement seemed exceptional. They were not huggers or kissers, and they never said, "I love you," to us that I remember. In college, everyone else seemed to end their phone conversations home with an "I love you," but I was too fearful of embarrassing my parents or making them uncomfortable ever to do that myself.

My father reminded us frequently that he was a "child of the Depression." He had grown up primarily in small towns in Indiana, and he was steeped in the Midwestern culture of self-reliance, which might explain his discomfort with expressions of affection. An only child of older parents, he was scarred by his mother's death from breast cancer in her mid-sixties and his father's almost self-directed death from congestive heart failure six months later. My father recognized that things don't always go well, and life can hit you with unpleasant surprises. He seemed to feel that you just had to keep going while keeping your fears and anxieties inside. He also was affected by his own strong faith. His father was a Methodist minister, and his mother a church organist, and he had attended divinity school for two years before deciding that his true calling was in journalism. I think his faith also informed his attitude of taking what comes and not assuming your problems are bigger or more important than anyone else's.

My mother's emotional distance was more of a modus operandi for her, not confined to moments of high stress, but characterizing all her interactions with others, including her family members. Her family was from Brunswick, Georgia, but she didn't live there until she was in high school in the mid-1940s, as her father served in a variety of capacities in U.S. embassies in Honduras, Guatemala, Cuba, and the Dominican Republic. I'm not sure if she learned to be detached because she moved a lot or if she loved moving a lot because she didn't develop relationships that made her regret leaving places. When my father "pinned" my mother in their senior year at Duke, her sorority sisters ran around asking each other which of her suitors had triumphed. She apparently managed to keep even her affection, or dare we call it love, for my father under wraps until she was forced to declare it. The early years of their marriage were apparently happy, but my mother withdrew emotionally after I was born, so their distance from each other is all I really knew. Somehow it translated into a very close family in which emotional suppression was the dominant characteristic.

One day, I confided to my sister how hurt and bewildered I was by our parents' behavior. She took the matter into her own hands, and at the next opportunity, she asked them why they weren't asking me how I was doing. I think they were surprised both at her directness and at my hurt. My mother said little; I wasn't particularly surprised. My father, on the other hand, acknowledged his, and perhaps even *their*, discomfort with expressing emotion and confronting unpleasant subjects. He spoke on behalf of my mother, knowing that I, via my sister Lucy, needed to hear that they both cared and knew they just weren't good at things like that.

For them, love was most comfortably expressed in action, in the myriad things they did for us and the amount of time they spent with us. We attended plays together, ate together every couple of weeks, saw each other every few days. My father attended almost every one of our children's sporting events. John told me after my diagnosis that my father had asked *him* some details about my situation. I'm sure he struggled with even that. After my father died, a friend told me that after my diagnosis, he had told her how brave he thought I was and how proud he was of me for my handling of the situation. Why didn't he ever tell me that? My rational self could understand why he might not ask me about specific details of my prognosis. I was stunned and hurt, however, that he could not summon up the courage to ask how I was doing when he saw me.

My mother could not acknowledge anyone's medical issues, including her own, and the only space in which she was comfortable expressing sentiment was about animals, particularly dogs. My sister and I were a bit jealous of the dogs, I think, because they were allowed to do anything they wanted: jump on the furniture, chew antiques, retrieve dirty balls that had been thrown against newly painted walls, remove plates from the kitchen counter to lick. If the dog limped for five minutes, my mother was at the vet. If the dog had had cancer, you can bet my mother would have done everything and asked it every day how it was. So, yes, I was resentful that my mother's attentions did not once fall on me.

Even in recent years as my parents declined physically and mentally and required more and more from me, I haven't managed to get over their reactions at the time. The hard-working, eager-to-please daughter, now gravely ill, was longing for a kind word and a bit of attention from my mother and father. Even as I started feeling hurt, I reminded myself that although they couldn't bring themselves to utter the words, they demonstrated their love by *doing* anything we needed. Our family's ability to get through my illness was made vastly easier by their loving *presence and actions*. During those many weeks, sitting in the infusion unit at Georgetown, I had some time to ruminate. I was grateful to know that Charlie and Emma were being well attended to, but hurt and angry that even my illness could not inspire some out-of-character parental tenderness.

But all these thoughts were not fully formed on that first day of chemotherapy. When it was time to leave, Mercedes gave me a list of instructions to follow over the next week, including the pills I was to take to suppress the likely nausea. She reminded me that I was going to face a greater risk of infection than normal because of the damage the chemotherapy was doing to my white blood cells. White blood cells fight infection, but because chemotherapy drugs kill off rapidly dividing cells such as hair, nails, the lining of various organs such as the nose, mouth, and stomach (and their main target, the cancer cells, one hopes), white blood cells are collateral damage but a not-so-easily lost part of the body.

I left that day with a laundry list of things I should do to avoid infection: Stay away from sick people (maybe stay away from non-family members altogether during my lowest point), stay away from public places, and don't eat fresh fruit or vegetables. John had warned me that oncology nurses give patients these draconian instructions, while oncologists tend to pooh-pooh them. I have never been a germophobe, and I have always been convinced that exposure to germs is healthy. Contrary to the prevailing ethos among parents in our community, my children were allowed to touch, yes, even eat things that had fallen on the floor. I did try to be more careful while I was on chemotherapy, recognizing that my body did not have its full defenses at the ready. But I didn't go into seclusion or stop eating fresh fruits and vegetables. I am probably lucky that I never developed an infection while on chemo, but I knew that eating canned peaches while quarantined was not going to be good for my health, either. The risk of depression trumped the risk of an infection.

When I was getting ready to leave the chemotherapy infusion unit that first day, Mercedes told me to return to Georgetown the next day to receive an injection of Neulasta, or pegfilgrastim, which is given about twenty-four hours after chemotherapy to counter the effects of the drugs by stimulating the production of "healthy" white blood cells in the bone marrow so as to boost the body's production of white blood cells and limit the weakening of the immune system.[1] Or that's the hope.

When I returned to the hospital the next day with John, the shot required only a quick visit of no more than ten minutes. As we sat there, the nurse casually said, "You know, Dr. Marshall, you could just give this to your wife at home. It's just a shot, and then you all wouldn't have to return to Georgetown for this." How could she have known that the last shot John ever gave was about fifteen years prior? After all, how hard could it be? He was a doctor!

---

1 "Neulasta," www. chemocare.com/chemotherapy/drug-info/Neulasta.aspx, September 14, 2019.

CHAPTER 12

The Wig
(As Liza Saw It)

I had long been an insider in the cancer world. I had heard so many personal stories from people with cancer or from caregivers and family members, ranging from world-famous athletes at the annual Lombardi Cancer Center Gala to people I didn't even know who found out that my husband was an oncologist and wanted to tell me *their* cancer story. Then I was diagnosed with the cancer that John publicly attacked on a regular basis. All of a sudden, I joined the breast cancer sorority, a group that I knew little about before my diagnosis but that now was sending me messages of support and giving me information, often from people I didn't know directly but who were connected with me through mutual friends.

At the top of the list of advice that breast cancer patients shared was dealing with impending hair loss. Through the newly discovered breast cancer network, a friend put me in touch with a friend of hers who was a bit further along in her breast cancer treatment. She told me that I should start the process of acquiring a wig as soon as I started chemotherapy so that I was ready when my hair started to come out.

She recommended a salon in Georgetown called Lucien Et Eivind as the place to go for the entire process, from selecting my "new hair" to shaving off what remained of my old locks. I wasn't sure about this at first. I knew our insurance would cover wigs and mastectomy bras and a breast prosthesis directly if I went to one of their approved distributors, which had revealing names such as Durable Medical Center and Nationwide Medical Supply. But when I called them, gruff men answered the phone, blandly informing me of their hours and services. They sounded completely indifferent to how a woman who had just undergone a mastectomy might feel.

Dr. Willey's nurse practitioner told me that Nordstrom had people who were certified in prosthesis and mastectomy bra fitting. When I called my insurance, they told me they would cover these items and a wig no matter who provided it; I would just have to do the paperwork myself. My love of paperwork has its limits, and insurance paperwork is one of those areas I would just as soon not have to do. I was willing to make an exception for the benefit of feeling like others when I was doing something that reminded me how different I now was.

At the salon, Hans handled cancer patients who were going to lose their hair. I had met him the week before at a Look Good Feel Better program at Georgetown. Look Good Feel Better is a nonprofit organization whose mission is to teach people with cancer ways to use cosmetics and accessories, such as wigs and scarves, to cover up the visible ravages of chemotherapy treatment, which frequently makes people look unwell. Pale and translucent skin, with no eyebrows and eyelashes (a new indignity that hadn't occurred to me until this program), can be tough to look at in the mirror. All over the United States, Look Good Feel Better holds free programs to teach people ways to draw eyebrows, experiment with scarves, use makeup options to counter the effects of cancer treatments on the skin, and so on. Plus, you walk away with swag, bags of cosmetics donated by cosmetic companies.

About two weeks after my surgery, I went to the main conference room at Lombardi, where I had attended baby showers for staff members. It was now set up like a classroom. Hans and the social worker who ran the program were upbeat as they greeted me and the other women. Mirrors on stands were perched on conference room tables, with chairs behind each mirror so that we faced the front of the room. Next to each mirror sat a cosmetic bag, its contents waiting to be discovered. Hans introduced himself to the ten women in attendance, and he described what was likely to happen to our skin and hair as we underwent cancer treatment, quickly followed by enthusiastic instruction on how to use the various makeup products to look good and feel better.

This was my first "getting together" with women who were going through what I was, and it was fun. I hadn't played with makeup in years, and the bag of goodies was overflowing with foundations, concealers, blushes, eye pencils, mascaras, and lipsticks. I felt like a teenager again. It was so nice to share stories with these women and to laugh at our inept attempts to put on makeup in a different way, never mind to tie scarves around our heads in something approaching attractive. We giggled as we missed with the eye pencils and literally tied our scarves in knots but not on our heads. Hans assured us that it would be much easier to handle the scarves when we didn't have hair. He made losing your hair sound appealing! Hans generously donated his time once a month to run the program at Georgetown, and he excelled at the job. He was humorous and knowledgeable, and he didn't treat us all as if we were delicate flowers or defective.

A week later, two days after my first chemotherapy treatment and on the first day of Charlie's and Emma's winter vacation, the whole family piled into the car and drove to the hair salon to select my new wig. I wasn't going to do that without everyone's approval. I wanted John to feel as comfortable as possible with how I looked during the next four to six months, and a fourteen-year-old boy and a ten-year-old girl can be brutal. I didn't want to embarrass the children any more than I was already with my high-waisted jeans and one breast (the former they had expressed, never the latter). Admittedly, Emma had suggested I get a blue mohawk wig, which I politely declined, so I wasn't sure how much help they were going to be.

Hans came out to greet us and took us back to a private area. He first showed us his wig room, where he must have had a hundred or more wigs, jauntily placed on Styrofoam heads. We oohed and aahed and started to whittle down the selection. I already had pretty short hair, and like my breast, I wasn't that attached to it. It wasn't great hair, part of the reason I kept it short. I had always envied other women's long, lush hair. As I thought about what I wanted to look like for the next six months or so, Hans cautioned that I didn't want to select a wig that was very different from my current hair. (The blue mohawk was out.) The goal, he said, is to preclude people from wondering what is going on, making it easier to go out, feel normal, and not have to tell every store clerk your medical history.

Hans placed me in a beauty salon chair in front of a mirror, and the fun began. Everyone had a ball. Being sick with cancer was not fun, but there were some moments of joy that I tried to hang onto. We went through quite a few sandy blond short-hair wigs until we settled on one that had a bit of spike to it. It looked mostly like me, but let me be a bit edgier than I was normally. Everyone enthusiastically approved it (maybe Mom would look a little cooler now), and Hans placed the order. I thought the wig looked sufficiently different from my own hair, but when I stopped wearing it five months later, as my hair was starting to come back in, but I was still obviously bald, several people I had seen regularly at church and school asked me what was going on. They hadn't noticed that I was wearing a wig or that I was undergoing chemotherapy at all! It was only when they saw my bald head that they realized something dramatic must have occurred.

Before we left Hans's salon, he suggested that as soon as I started to lose my hair in a few weeks, I should come back to let him shave it off. He had observed that women found it upsetting to wake up each morning to find chunks of hair on their pillows and that shaving it all off then could make things easier.

In late December, just before New Year's Day, I woke up one morning to find the anxiously anticipated clump of hair on my pillow. As I shampooed, pieces of hair plastered my wet hands. I had known it was coming, but it was still a shock to see my hair falling out. I choked up as I tried to rinse the hair off my hands. I then emerged from the shower and said dejectedly to John, "I guess it's time to see Hans."

On January 3, the day after my second round of chemotherapy, I returned with some trepidation to Hans's special room for the removal of my hair. I didn't ask anyone to go with me. John was back at work, and Charlie and Emma had returned to school after the holidays. I was pretty sure I could handle this one alone. Hans asked me if I wanted to watch him shave my head, which was considerate, but I declined. He turned me with my back to the mirror and gently removed all of my hair with an electric razor. It was an odd sensation; I'd never thought about shaving my head before I got cancer. I steeled myself for the turn back, and he revolved the chair so that I faced the mirror. It wasn't so bad. I had wanted edgy, and I definitely had that now. And I had a wig, which he showed me how to put on and care for. One of the big choices in the wig realm is whether to get real human hair or synthetic hair. My friends who had been through chemo recommended the synthetic because such wigs are much cheaper and hold their shape and condition much better than those of human hair. It felt prickly and odd, but it looked pretty real, and I was satisfied with the way I looked even if it was suddenly so different.

I picked the kids up from school and received rave reviews. I was glad I had included them in the selection. That night I took the wig off so everyone could see my bald head. Emma wanted to draw on it as they had drawn on the head of a teacher at school who had had breast cancer, but I refused the offer. The kids clearly enjoyed my new look and didn't seem at all uncomfortable about it. John enthused about how sexy and cute I looked. I kind of liked it, too. It's fascinating to see your head without hair, with every bump and freckle that have gone unseen all your life finally revealed. The next morning, I got up, showered, rubbed some shampoo on as Hans had recommended to keep my scalp moisturized, rinsed it off, and dressed. No need to dry, style, rub hair products in. I put the wig on and was good to go.

Even as the wig became part of my look, I never felt completely normal in it. I always knew it wasn't the real me. And yet it did make me *appear* to be relatively normal, forestalling questions about my health and curious glances from strangers and friends. But as the day wore on, it grew uncomfortable: Some hair in the front constantly hung over my eyes, and my scalp got itchy and sweaty. When I was home, I didn't wear it unless I was expecting someone. Sometimes I would even take it off when non-family members were there. Occasionally the children would have a friend visiting, and I would hear them approaching the room I was in. I felt I needed to warn them that I was not wearing the wig, so I would yell, "Top down!" Charlie or Emma would say casually to their friend, "My mom isn't wearing her wig. Do you want to see?" The friend would enter the room, hesitant and wide-eyed, to see what I looked like and then depart satisfied. Those experiences always made me smile. Being bald, at least temporarily, wasn't always a bad thing.

CHAPTER 13

The Wig
(As John Saw It)

After delivering the terrible news of the diagnosis, the next order of business for oncologists is to describe the treatment and its side effects. Cancer cells and normal cells share one essential characteristic: many normal cells are dependent on dividing, too, and are therefore vulnerable to chemo. Blood cells, skin cells, the lining of the mouth, the GI tract, and (for many, the scariest of all) hair cells are constantly replaced, requiring new cells to be made 24/7. Yet many of the more miserable and dangerous side effects of chemo— reducing the bone marrow cells to the point you cannot fight an infection, leaving behind mouth sores so painful it hurts to eat, or having severe dehydrating diarrhea from killing the lining of your GI tract— seem to diminish in importance to our attachment to our hair.

Oncologists are trained to list the more life-threatening and permanent side effects first because they scare *us* the most. But the whole time we are going through our sometimes-horrifying list, we can see the anticipatory fear in the eyes of the patient, the unsaid really big question hanging in the room. Not "Will this poison work?" Or "Is there any way to reduce the side effects?" Or "Is this all worth it?" The really big question is "Will I lose my hair?" Over the years I learned to start there since there are two easy answers: "Yes, you will" or "No, you probably won't." Let's get it over with so that the patient will listen to the serious parts. But as soon as we suggest hair loss, the tension in the room increases. You see the wince followed by brief glances full of sadness and pity exchanged by the patient and the partner. The brave, stiff-upper-lip types offer the philosophical response of "Who needs hair anyway?" Many sink in their seats, visibly pained. Strangely, men's reactions are often stronger than those of women. Women understand wigs and reconcile themselves to the fact they will end up wearing one. There is no rule preventing men from wearing a wig, but let's be honest, they really shouldn't, and thank God, they almost never do.

Some of our patients have said, "I will do anything you ask except take drugs that cause hair loss. I would rather be dead." Or "I cannot stand the thought of being in my coffin at my funeral with no hair!" We do everything we can to depathologize hair loss, to prevent patients from drawing a line in the sand that they will regret. We introduce them to other patients who have lost hair and survived. We refer them to wig shops, websites, anything that might dissuade them from opting for their sometimes life-endangering ultimatum. We occasionally lose the argument and use therapies that do not cause hair loss even if that can mean a significantly inferior outcome.

A lot of the breast cancer drugs cause all the mature hair all over the body to come out, interestingly replaced by a fine, soft down of baby hair. Many other chemo treatments cause enough of the hair to come out so everyone will notice: uneven thinning, patches of baldness on one spot, still some hair on others. Many patients cling to their last few wisps of hair. (Maybe I sympathize with the strategy since it resembles the way that I am clinging to mine.) They hide their baldness under a baseball cap or a scarf, or buy big floppy hats that they wear everywhere.

I try to explain that wearing a business suit and a baseball cap is fooling no one. "Cut it off!" I want to yell. "This is your chance! You will look so very cool, so hot. Let your cancer flag fly!" This is the time to get one or both ears pierced. Or get a tattoo on the back of your scalp. (I would suggest one that says, "Cancer sucks.") When you find that first clump of hair on your pillow or in the shower, cut it very short, thus sparing the emotionally scaring moment when the last strands fall out. Think of the big shave as a fresh start, not an end.

One of our family's fondest memories during our entire breast cancer chapter was wig shopping. Liza tried on some new looks: blond, brunette, metallic, spiky, flowing. The kids and Liza seemed to be having a really good time, with smiles of joy all around. I was not sharing in the joy, and I tried to hide it. I was not going to dampen the high spirits this time, but with every wig, every modeling walk down the runway, I saw Liza not with a fresh, hip look, her wig not as a prop to prevent the unavoidable public stares from strangers.

I saw Liza as being really sick.

Even though I have spent my professional life reassuring patients about being bald and extolling the glories of wigs for women, I am painfully aware of their shortcomings. Wigs never fit quite right. You almost always can tell that someone is wearing one, but like the socially risky question "Are you pregnant?," you never can ask. As patients go through chemo, most lose weight, their faces thin, they become pale, and the wig gets looser and looser, slipping around and needing constant adjustment. Some patients insist on wearing their wigs every-where, determined never to be seen bald. Some patients lie dying in a hospital bed and insist on wearing their wig, now so loose that it stays fixed to the pillow as the patient turns her head to greet you. As I watched Liza try on the next new look, I remembered my mom's wigs. I remembered the look of all the patients melting away in front of me, wearing a wig that had become an inadequate reminder of their former self, now half covering their eyes.

When Liza tried on the next wig, all I could see was her dying.

Liza and the kids broke into my darkness, asking, "What do you think of this one?"

"I love it!" I answered.

CHAPTER 14

Love at First Sight

John and I met over a beer keg at a fraternity party on October 3, 1981. I was an eighteen-year-old sophomore and he was a twenty-year-old junior at Duke University.

Honestly, it was love at first sight. This tall, lanky young man with curly brown hair, wearing a yellow button-down shirt and a beat-up navy-blue sweater, stood on the other side of a circle of people, exuding confidence, humor, and warmth. He smiled at me, his eyes twinkling with a certain mischief, and we started talking. He was from Lexington, Kentucky. He asked where I was from, and I said, "Alexandria, Virginia. You've probably never heard of it." "Actually, I went to high school there," he replied. In fact, we had gone to high school across the street from each other, I to the public high school and he to a private all-boys boarding school. We quickly discovered that both of our mothers had had cancer.

He had been raised in the South in the 1960s and 1970s, so he had a few sexist attitudes, but I was delighted to meet a man who didn't view my intelligence, ambition, and independence as a threat. In fact, he seemed to delight in them and to be proud of me and my accomplishments. He was unabashed about enjoying things others might find feminine. He cooked, he cleaned, he dressed in things other than jeans and T-shirts, he could express his emotions (a welcome change from my family experience), and he was loving and caring. What I thought and said mattered to him.

Fortunately for me, love at first sight was mutual. John always told anyone who would listen that he was in a bad place when we met and that he had prayed the night before we met to find someone to help him turn his life around. (In fact, he's probably told you already.) I think I had always been ready to find someone, and John seemed perfect. (He isn't, but he's pretty close.) We never dated anyone else after we met, and we planned to get married as soon as I graduated from college, despite each of us being taken aside by our own parents for a serious conversation to dissuade us from such an early marriage. But we were in love, and we didn't want to live apart, even though neither of us had a job or any certain plans after my graduation.

John, who graduated from Duke in three years in order to save his family money, had been working hard to get into medical school, taking classes at the University of Kentucky to improve his academic record. His first two years of college grades were not impressive, so he had some ground to make up. As my graduation and our wedding approached in 1984, we decided that we would apply to medical schools and law schools in mostly the same places in hopes of being able to attend school and live together at the same time. That was not to be, so just after our June wedding, when I was twenty-one and John was twenty-three, he started medical school at the University of Louisville. Meanwhile, I deferred my admission to the University of Virginia Law School for three years and worked in Louisville to support us.

All of our decisions obviously worked out, despite our parents' trepidation, and we built a solid marriage and family, settling with our dog in Arlington, Virginia, after my graduation from law school. We thrived in two demanding careers for several years until Charlie was born. I then tapered down my job with a law firm in Washington, D.C., and after Emma was born, I worked from home about fifteen hours a week. After eight years, I quit and became what I liked to call a "professional volunteer." My roles included deacon and elder at church, room mother and member of the Board of Trustees at school, and Brownie "cookie mom." Also, I was a founding board member for the local chapter of a cancer support organization called The Wellness Community at the time, now Hope Connections for Cancer Support.

One major reason that I reduced my work and eventually stopped is that John's career was blossoming. He was invited to speak across the country and around the world on the subject of gastrointestinal cancers and the development of new treatments. He consulted with pharmaceutical companies on new cancer drugs, which involved more travel. I decided that I no longer could be tied to private law firm demands and hours. It was a sacrifice I felt I needed to make for the family, but it did change the dynamics of our marriage. I was no longer earning money, which meant all the income was John's. Few people sought me out at parties to talk about my work, and when they did ask me, I would mumble that I was a stay-at-home mom who did a lot of volunteer work. However, everyone wanted to talk to John. They didn't quite push past me, but it was clear that he was the star attraction, not just because he worked, and I didn't, but because he is funny, engaging, and charismatic.

John has an incisive and mischievous sense of humor. He loves to be provocative, which frequently works well for him even if it makes those around him uncomfortable. He can make fun of a total stranger, and they smile warmly! And engage! Most people would get punched or at least given a baleful stare. The topics he picks to tease people can be controversial, designed not only to get a laugh but also to puncture a few cherished notions about issues he might understand better—for instance, healthcare.

John's love of attention first manifested itself with his childhood dream of being a Broadway musical star. He has regaled me with stories of his school performances, singing in his good tenor all the words to *his* songs as well as many others in the Broadway musical canon. He has turned his remarkable stage presence into excellent public speaking, and he has gone on the road almost every week to give a talk somewhere. His humor also causes his patients to adore him as he treats them with warmth and jokes about their biggest fears, bringing them into the open.

When you live with a man one of my friends dubbed "Mr. Personality," and when his career is skyrocketing, and when you have given up your own career to support his, your self-esteem can take a hit. In the years before I was diagnosed with breast cancer, John and I started having occasional battles about how he prioritized his family and his home life. While he would tell me periodically that he'd be glad to stay home and have me go back to work, I think he would have died a slow death in that role. I used to joke that his speaking engagements combined my two greatest fears: flying on planes and public speaking. But for John, the travel and the attention were his lifeblood. By the time I was diagnosed with breast cancer, I think neither one of us felt the other truly appreciated the work we were doing or the sacrifices we were making to support each other's desires and the family's needs. Maybe a breast cancer diagnosis was what we needed to learn to appreciate each other again.

Unfortunately, the type of cancer I got is John's Mortal Enemy Number One. Breast cancer actually might get more attention than he does. One of the biggest platforms on John's bully pulpit when he addresses groups of people in the field of oncology, from pharmaceutical companies and cancer care advocates to private practicing oncologists and academics, is his "hatred" of breast cancer. I put that in quotation marks because I'm not sure he really *hates* it, but he does come pretty close. It's not the disease, but the pink ribbons and the runs for the cure and the money that results from those marketing devices. John's talks long have included a few minutes of ranting when he asks why breast cancer gets ten times the funding received by all other cancers combined. This part understandably is not always well-received. I have heard women talking in the bathroom after one of his talks with dismay and high dudgeon about what he said about breast cancer. How could he say that?! Doesn't he care about women with breast cancer? Easy for him to say, *he'll* never get it. He has been called out by audience members at his talks, but he is unfazed.

You'd think John's stance would bother me, too. That's the disease that threatens to kill me, destroy our family, take me away from you. Don't you want everything to be thrown at finding a cure, mitigating the side effects of treatment, preventing your children and grandchildren from getting it? But I didn't feel that way at all.

I recognize that my life and those of all breast cancer patients aren't the only ones that matter. They certainly do matter, but so do those of bone cancer patients and brain cancer patients and, particularly for John, gastrointestinal cancer patients. I've met many of John's patients and their families; we frequently are approached by people John has treated or their surviving family members. I think I have a pretty good sense of their desperation to see advances in the treatment of *their* cancers and how frustrating it must be when the only cancer that gets a ribbon on the White House and pink cleats and towels for a whole month in the NFL is breast cancer. John *should* speak up for *his* patients and for *their* diseases; he should call out the fact that all other cancers are significantly underfunded compared with breast cancer, a community that I think has somewhat lost its way.

Myriad illnesses afflict people all over the world, and I have no reason to believe that my illness or my cure is any more important than those. Perhaps there is no solution to this problem, but I am glad that John is bringing attention to it, and if he needs to call attention to the "breast cancer machine," I support that, too. Perhaps that machine could channel some resources for the development of advocacy and fundraising skills in other cancers and other deadly and debilitating illnesses. I know I'm a dreamer.

CHAPTER 15

Caregiver 1.0

We had been married for twenty-two years when Liza was diagnosed with breast cancer. We had made all the kids we were going to make. My vasectomy was the best $60 I ever spent, since it also marked the end of birth control pills for Liza. (We wouldn't want to increase her risk of cancer, for goodness' sake.) We had settled into our respective lives and roles: mine to make the money; Liza's to manage us all. We each had our own focus and our own set of priorities. Sometimes these priorities overlapped, but often they did not. Liza read the sports section every day; I read the obits. Liza prioritized exercise; I had no time to work out. Every morning I left Liza and the kids to go off to work, deal with cancer, manage the operation of a complex division, and have meetings all day long. Liza saw it as that I "got to" go off to work, talk to adults, and have a break from parenting. We saw the other's life as the better one, the more interesting one, the easier one.

A simmering, rarely discussed mutual resentment had developed between us. Maybe this is just a stage all married people go through as the years march along. I felt as if I was working very hard, dutifully engaged in a difficult, emotionally and physically taxing job. Liza was taking kids to school, running fundraisers, giving our money to worthy causes, and finding tickets for the best shows. Sure, I might have traveled, but I always caught crazy flights back, adding to my stress, to make sure I got home for the show, for the kid's recital, or just to get home. Liza saw my travel as a chance to escape, see new places, meet new people, and dine at new restaurants.

I put in long hours, talked too much about work, and was visibly stressed. I was completely dedicated to the family, and my career choices were easily justified as being done ultimately for them. No boys' nights out, no golf outings. I was driven, and Liza was equally driven. Our relationship had fallen into a routine, predictable and on the verge of boring. (I hate being boring.) Everything we did was for the collective good, but rarely did we do something special for each other. We were a fabulous team: full-time partners, romance less of a priority. Nothing much was going to change for us, not until the kids left the house, when I retired, or when one of us died.

As I looked at my patients, I've often thought that it is much harder to be the caregiver than the patient. Having surgery and chemo sucks, but as a recompense, the patient gets attention, gifts, days off work, naps, drugs, greeting cards, and a lot of people asking how you are. All eyes are on the patient, and all prayers are directed her way. The kids get a few nods and a few expressions of concern, but typically the caregiver is left out in the emotional cold. Plus, caregivers get more work, less sleep, no get-well cards, and no attention. The essential yet invisible caregivers are the pit crew for the race car driver, the caddy to the golfer, and the camera man to the star. No one notices you when things go well, but everyone blames you when things go wrong. Caregiving is not a good fit for me.

That's not even the worst of it! In cases where the patient's cancer is terminal, the caregiver role becomes a full-time job, particularly in the last six months or so of life. Being the "end of life" caregiver might be the hardest job of all, a transition to a non-stop, twenty-four-hour maintenance of another's life. Imagine having a helpless newborn but without any of the joy of growth and development, never any positive milestones, just steady decline. Pain, weakness, weight loss (as the caregiver gains weight, eating all the uneaten food lovingly made in hopes the patient would just eat a little), not enough strength to go out, sleeping through birthday dinners, not coming down for Christmas, events scheduled as celebrations of life becoming only reminders of loss. This person you are caring for is your life's partner, your entire world. You cannot imagine a world without her, but in many ways, she is already gone.

When Liza dies of her cancer, all I can imagine is that I will have to remain alive, reminded every day of my irreplaceable life partner. I will have lost the person sent by God to help be my rudder and my conscience. I have watched too many surviving spouses try to go on after the loss of a spouse to cancer, adjusting to the abrupt transition from caregiver to widow or widower. Some try to create a totally new life, maybe reinvent themselves, but many are lost, wandering alone for their remaining days. Inevitably I saw myself as a lonely wanderer.

In the long list of my deficiencies is caregiving. My family will attest that I have little interest in their cold, stomach ache, fever, or bruised knee. A deep cut requiring stitches will get my attention but little compassion. Anything less than a life-threatening, major illness bores me. There is a good reason that I did not stay with primary care.

Why waste my valuable skills and time on minor ailments, most of which doctors do nothing for? Even when my patients ask about flu shots, blood pressure, diabetes, concern over a mole, I really don't care unless it somehow interferes with treating their cancer. Let their caregiver worry about those things—I don't have the time, patience, or bandwidth. In reality, I do actually care, but if I cannot do much about it except hold your hand and be there, I will disappoint. I am terrible at hand-holding and giving emotional support. After thirty seconds of quiet, I get uncomfortable and restless, then try to make a joke or ask an inappropriate question. I feel an expectation to entertain, and failing that, I check my watch and phone, pick up a magazine, and finally resort to entertaining myself.

Sadly, I treat my family worse than any patient, any acquaintance from church, anyone. The family has given up on me for day-to-day attention. When it comes to family illness, I lose perspective and objectivity. The family assumes that having a doctor in the family is useful, sort of a medical Swiss Army knife. When they come to me with an ailment, and I run through the possible "differential diagnoses" in my head, as all good doctors do, instead of common, likely possibilities, I can conjure only sure-to-be terminal illnesses. If Emma has a fever, it must be leukemia. If Charlie's hip hurts after a soccer game, it must be an osteosarcoma. If the dog has runny bowels for a few days, it is certainly canine colon cancer.

When Liza was diagnosed, and her first mastectomy was just a few days ahead, one of my first thoughts was that she could die from just the surgery. Mind you, while I am truly an optimist, I know that in any operation where general anesthesia is used, fractions of a percentage point of people die. Sure, one in one hundred thousand is rare, but someone has to be the "one," and that someone could be Liza. Naturally, as a highly skilled and organized man, I panicked. I had no idea where she kept her log-ins for the computer or the bank. How does she pay our bills, and has she paid the bills? I had never focused on running our household because this was her domain. Regularly reminded that I would never do it right anyway, I associated household administration with emotionally damaging failure. I could see the path ahead. Every accounting corner I cut, every missed entry into the almighty Quicken, would cause her immeasurable distress and more nausea than the chemo. The chaos would be shared with me, making us both so tense with my incompetence that she would want her cancer to grow faster to put her out of her misery. I needed a lesson in Household 101, and I needed one quickly.

Liza agreed. We set aside time before her surgery for her to take me through it all.

Liza began her instructions: "Here is where I keep passwords. You will have to memorize them and then eat the paper they are written on."

There were nearly one hundred passwords, with no real patterns, bizarre strings of n0Mb3Rs and LeTteRz, different for each account. No one will ever hack into our world, including me.

She continued faster than I could either take notes or remember. "Here is how to log into the bank. Here is how to see your paycheck; here is how to make sure it is right; here is how I pay the bills; and please do it my way. Here is where I keep the kids' records and all our important documents. Here is where we keep the rest of the important documents. Here is my safety deposit key—Where is yours?"

Beads of sweat appear on my forehead. I have no idea where my key is. There is only one place I ever keep things like this, but I have zero memory of ever putting it there. I go to my secret drawer, and in my secret box, where I keep my one and only password for everything, there is a key that looks like Liza's. I stop, look up, and thank God. In the stress of the fear of the lost key, I had forgotten everything she just told me and already swallowed the paper with all the passwords on it. If Liza dies, we are doomed.

I needed to step up my game and reprioritize. Liza will be first, the kids second, job third, anything remaining of my life last. There will be even less time for exercise, travel, late meetings, and dinners out. Hopefully this would be a short-term problem. Surgery, then chemo for a few months, then back to normal. At least that is the process, the desired path, the hoped-for outcome my patients hear me describe every day. Just get through this phase, but then back to normal.

Of course, I knew this was not going to be for just a few months.

Some basic caregiver fundamentals I was sure of. I had to stay healthy. I had to stay employed. The health insurance came from my work, and we needed the money to pay for the house, schools, food, cars, and heat. Did I have to slow down at work? A lot of people counted on me—our staff, our patients, my adoring fans. Would slowing down even a little reverse my hard-earned gains to finding a cure for cancer? Putting off any real decisions, I fired off a few e-mails to warn that I might have to cancel my appearance at a few scheduled trips. My clinic schedule was booked for the next two months. If Liza received treatment at Georgetown, then I could keep the work balls in the air while being there for her.

In any relationship, there is a natural, almost rhythmic flow of energy, karma, back and forth, the yin and the yang of life. Through life, there are periods when the flow of support is one-directional, like studying for the medical boards or the bar exam, pregnancy, a rough patch at work, difficulty with a friend or a child. Most of our lives together, I think a lot of the flow had been in my favor, living around me and my needs. In the inevitable regression to the mean, this was going to be a payback time.

When cancer invades a house, whatever skeletons are hiding in the closet rattle louder. I have seen many couples break apart, under too much stress for an already fragile relationship. Sexual interest falls, added burdens are placed on everyone, and sacrifices must be made, often with unspoken resentment. Inside you are screaming, "How dare she get cancer? How dare cancer screw up our lives, impose upon my happiness, disrupt our established order, interfere with my career, take away the joy of our love life?!" Certainly I could not say that to her, our friends, her friends, and definitely the children. I had not yet discovered therapy, so no outlet there. I just had to take it, bottle it up, and add it to the miasma within.

I was not sure I had it in me. I am selfish. I need attention and expressions of affection. I need my batteries charged all the time. I need to look forward to things. Liza and I were stable but no longer exciting. She would be unable to provide what I needed, so I would either have to go without or fulfill my needs in other ways. I think about all of my patients, all the stories I have heard, all the couples I know who split up during cancer. This is not really about sex, although sex is important. It is more about affection and support flowing only one way. The patient needs a lot and can return only a fraction. At least that is how the caregiver feels, real or perceived. Liza and I already had mutual resentment brewing, and maybe it could rip us apart should the flow run mostly one way for long.

I needed to show everyone that I not only could talk the talk, but also walk the walk. As a caring cancer doctor, I should be perfect for the job! I know everything there is to know about cancer, chemo, side effects, and expectations. I have years of experience guiding patients and families as they travel their own cancer journey; I coach them through rough spots; I offer proven strategies to deal with their kids. I had been in training for this role all my life. "Liza is so lucky to have you on her side," everyone said to me. "With John by your side, you all will be just fine," everyone said to Liza. To us both, "You guys are already such pros at this; we know you will be fine."

So it was no big deal when I got the assignment of giving Liza a subcutaneous shot of Neulasta, a medicine to shorten the time her blood counts were low after chemo. We ask patients and caregivers to give subcutaneous shots all the time. They are easy, and most of the time our nurses train them, overseeing the first shot to make sure that patients and caregivers get it right. Sometimes, especially when the patients have given shots before or if the caregivers are medical people, we skip the training. There's no need to waste our time or the patient's time. All that's needed is a quick conversation about any special instructions and a bit of reassurance that this will be a breeze.

I am a real physician, so even though I had not given anyone a subcutaneous shot in the past decade, I knew the ropes. I had never given a Neulasta shot to anyone, though, and I received no training from our nurses since they assumed I knew. I probably told them I had it under control since I've prescribed this stuff hundreds of times. Despite the fact we were in uncharted territory here, giving a shot was definitely something that I could do well.

The moment of truth was upon us that evening. We were in our bathroom, the location of all major medical procedures in our house. The kids wanted to watch, but we asked them to stay out for now. They lurked outside in the hall. I got the Neulasta out of the fridge and took the syringe out of the box. I took a quick look to make sure that it was the right drug, the right dose, meant for Liza—standard, best-practice stuff. I found the spot on her arm and applied a little alcohol to her skin. Liza braced for the worst, needle in, Neulasta injected quickly to get it over with. Immediately, Liza let out a loud shriek of pain, frightening to even the neighbors who likely called the police to report the crime. The kids ran in. "WHAT HAPPENED??" Liza was crying. Through her tears, she gave me a glare that only an angry wife can produce. The bathroom was getting crowded with all the people and all the rage. I decided it would be a good idea for incompetent me to leave.

The next morning, I walked up to the infusion unit where Liza was being treated, head hung low. Mercedes, Liza's main nurse and a good friend of mine, knew immediately what had happened. Mercedes asked in a reproachful tone, "Dr. Marshall, you did not know how to give that shot, did you?"

"I thought I did," I replied, embarrassed (make that humiliated).

"Did you allow the shot to get to room temperature?"

"No."

"Did you give it slowly?"

"No."

"Did you read the instructions?"

"No."

Shaking her head in disgust, Mercedes sat me down and gave me the lesson I had declined the day before. After about a week, Liza forgave me. I started to read the directions. I gave the remaining doses with humility and care, just as I had been instructed. As I have said, I often use our family's stories in my lectures, and the shot story instantly became a regular feature in my medical road show. I told my patients and their families. Every time I prescribed a shot "to go," I told the story again. I told our fellows as part of their training. I needed to share how my doctor's arrogance hurt my own wife. I needed to share the importance of sweating the small stuff so that others would not suffer as Liza had. I needed to remind myself of how complex and disruptive our treatments are for our patients. And I needed to remind myself of how a little extra time to describe a simple thing like a shot could make someone else's night a little smoother.

CHAPTER 16

Last Christmas

I had my first round of chemotherapy on December 18, and then came Christmas. This was starting to look even sadder than Thanksgiving as I was going to be at my low point a week after my first chemotherapy, which would coincide with Christmas Day. My parents and sister already had planned a Christmas trip because the four of us had planned to be in Kentucky, and they had not wanted to celebrate Christmas at home alone.

Now it was going to be just the four of *us* at home alone for the holidays with the sword of Damocles as our guest. We struggled with the change of plans and decided that we all needed and even deserved something special. Was this going to be my last Christmas with my family? That thought was both impossible to avoid and impossible to dwell on. I couldn't help but remember that John had been wrong when he had assured Holly that the first Christmas after her diagnosis wouldn't be her last. Damn it, if it were going to be my last, it was going to be a good one. So we made a reservation for

Christmas dinner at the fanciest restaurant in town, Citronelle, run by renowned chef Michel Richard.

After a morning of opening gifts and an afternoon of playing with them, plus a nap and the requisite viewing of *A Charlie Brown Christmas*, Charlie and John put on their best suits and ties while Emma and I were attired in our most elegant dresses, and we drove into the center of Georgetown, marveling at the glittering lights on houses and shops along the way. The restaurant felt inviting, with its own greenery and twinkling white lights brightening the dark room and the warmth of light and heat emanating from the open kitchen. It was an evening of pure joy and indulgence as we laughed and chatted while relishing one delectable dish after another. The famed Michel Richard even invited the kids into the kitchen to watch them cook. It was one of our most memorable holidays, not because it was sad, but because it was happy and loving and festive in ways that felt so intimate, so authentic to our family.

But was it going to be my last? At some point I would have to confront the fact that I *might* be dead by next Christmas…or the one after that…or sometime before my children were grown, and John was too old to remarry, and I viewed myself as actually *old* enough to die. I had many thoughts about all of that during the period between my diagnosis and my surgery, partly because it was all so new then and partly because I was just as concerned about dying under anesthesia as I was about the cancer getting me. I was scared. I didn't mind the thought of dying at some point, but this was much too soon. Going through the various phases of treatment, I had plenty of time to think about dying. When I was in the infusion unit or the Lombardi clinic waiting room, I saw people who were on their last desperate treatment, barely able to get through but determined not to concede.

I'm a pragmatist, preferring not to see things through rose-colored glasses. I find that preparing for the worst helps me. I am very good at imagining terrible things happening to me or to people I love, so in a sense, when people die, I may have already completed my mourning. I didn't cry at Holly's funeral or my mother-in-law's, but I had cried when it became clear that they were *going* to die. I accept death as part of life and know that it comes to some people sooner than others.

But if I say that out loud, the person I am addressing is usually shocked. I have assured everyone that I don't want to live to the point at which I can no longer do the things I enjoy. I think that in the United States, we have an unhealthy relationship with death. We fight and fight and expect everyone else to fight and fight no matter how unpleasant and exhausting that fight is. Not everyone wants to fight.

Part of my relative calm regarding death is my faith, which does help, but like many people of faith, I have times of doubt. Then the pragmatist reappears: I won't know anything when I'm dead, so why does it matter to me? My real concern, of course, is for those I leave behind, starting with John. During my treatment, we never verbalized the fact that there was a real possibility of my death, but I imagine he thought about it a lot. With the experience of a mother dying of cancer, it was not difficult to replace images of her with images of me being sick, lying in a hospital bed, a shadow of my former self. And he could put himself in the place of his father, trying to keep it all together, making sure that the children were happy and getting on with their lives, and caring for an ailing and gradually dying wife.

I didn't want my children to grow up without their mother. Through John's experience, I had some idea of what that was like, to experience joys in life—such as graduation, a new job, a wedding, an achievement, having children—without one of your parents to share the joy, pride, and excitement with you. Also, you needed to be able to go to them for advice as you experience challenges in life. Even though John and his brother and sister were fortunate enough to have a wonderful stepmother—who essentially *became* their mother not long after their mother was gone—regrets and sadness still appear from not having *their* mother with them as they grew up and experienced the highs and lows of life.

I also didn't want my family to go through the ordeal of watching me decline, knowing I was going to die. I didn't want them to be sad or lonely. Heck, my parents' sadness was so profound that they couldn't even *acknowledge* my cancer. People aren't supposed to die in their forties. Children aren't supposed to die before their parents. Parents aren't supposed to die before becoming grandparents.

And then we come back to the fact that, for purely selfish reasons, I didn't want to die. I was forty-three years old. I wanted to see my children grow up, where they were going to go to high school and college, what they were going to study, whom they were going to marry, what they were going to name their kids. I had a lot of opinions that still needed to be expressed and advice that needed to be given. I didn't want to leave.

I have come to realize that no matter how sanguine you are about the concept of death, confronting it is an entirely different matter. My parents have helped me experience this more fully in the past few years as they have aged and have been forced to grapple with more and more medical issues. It increasingly became clear that they were both ready to go. And yet, months before he died, I sat with my father in the emergency room after he had had some "episode." I could see the fear in his eyes, and the tears roll down his cheeks as he realized that might be it. He was a man of deep faith, coping with the debilitation of a stroke, and he clearly felt that his life was largely frustrating and boring and not worth the effort. But he too wanted to see his grandchildren grow up and maybe see *their* children. He wanted to witness and participate in everything that is yet to come.

My only defense against all of these existential realities was not to think about it. Yes, we all learn that repression and denial are not good things, but for me they were essential emotional protections that became healthy responses to an irreducibly terrifying and depressing situation. I believe that faith is more than just a mechanism to give comfort in the face of a terrifying and depressing world. I believe in God because I see and feel God around me almost every day. So I did my best to put my trust in God, not that I believed God would personally intervene to save me because I was so special. My faith helped me to accept that whatever happened to me and to my family, God would be there. That knowledge somehow freed me to proceed by just putting one foot in front of the other. There was so much about my life that I loved, and I couldn't see the point in ruining those moments and those realities by dwelling on the awful things that might be yet to come. I didn't want to ruin everyone else's days either. Charlie and Emma *didn't* need to be mourning their mother before she was gone, and John's hands were full trying to care for everyone. For our family and for me personally, I didn't want to spend my time being sad and afraid.

Early on in my treatment, I visited a psychiatrist who specializes in breast cancer patients. I wasn't sure if I needed help, and I had never seen a therapist before, but I didn't want to mess this up. So I found my way to her office one day, noting a box of tissues on every surface. ("So I'm supposed to cry here," I thought.) She was wonderful and talked the basics through with me. I returned a second time, and halfway through the session, she said, in essence, that she didn't think I needed therapy. She went on to say that her experience is that people who are sad with their lives make big changes after they have breast cancer, but that people who are happy with their lives generally continue as they were despite a breast cancer diagnosis. That was me.

It is also true that confronting death makes you appreciate what is right in front of you. Kind of like that Christmas. Life *is* short, for everyone. Few people are really *ready* to die when they do. There is always more to see and to do. But the only way to enjoy life is to be present. So in that way, being under the threat of an earlier death than you had planned can be seen, without too much of a stretch, as a bit of a blessing.

People would tell me how sorry they were about my cancer, and I would say with complete sincerity, "Well, it's better than being hit by a bus." I meant it. If I were to die from my breast cancer, I was going to prepare myself, to prepare my family, to say good-byes, to write that letter to the kids. I remember sitting with Holly one day as she was nearing the end, but fretting about her son and his homework. We commiserated about getting our kids to do their homework, and I realized that all Holly wanted to worry about was whether her son was going to do what he needed to do in school. For all of us, these worries were privileges and not burdens. To stay alive to deal with the crap was worth it because it meant you are alive to enjoy the parts of life that *aren't* crap, the moments and even extended periods of beauty and joy.

After our Christmas dinner at Citronelle, merry and sated, we drove home, a bit quieter than we had driven into town. Charlie, who even at fourteen displayed a precocious talent for food and drink, led us in a deconstruction of his dessert, a Michel Richard specialty, Breakfast Surprise. It looked like a boiled egg, sausage, bacon, and hash browns, but it really was composed of chocolate, custard, and other sweets. We talked about what we wanted to do during the rest of the winter holiday. Planning the future, even for just a few days, was reassuring. However happy and calm I was, the thought that this might be my last Christmas or that I might be much less able to celebrate it next year was never far from my mind.

When we arrived home, we sat around the tree, admiring our handiwork in selecting it, decorating it, and keeping the needles on it. We slowly drifted upstairs and put on our new Christmas pajamas. I read a bit with Emma, as we always did, and John chatted with Charlie before we kissed them both good night. "I think that was a good Christmas, don't you?" I asked. John smiled and put his arms around me and held me tight. "Yes," he said quietly, "the best."

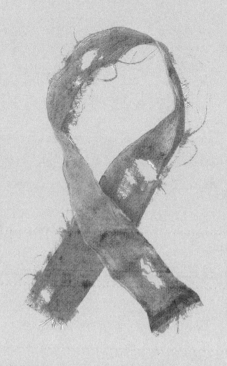

PART 4

Gifts

Fellows' noon lecture series: Doctor/Patient Interactions
Georgetown University
Washington, D.C.
August 2009

I want to check in on how the year is going so far, making sure things are going smoothly, particularly for you first-years. We sometimes forget what a big transition it is from being an internal medicine resident to a hematology-oncology fellow. It's an even bigger deal for those of you who are new to Georgetown. So keep thinking about issues you want to discuss, concerns you have with patients, our faculty, the call schedule—whatever comes to mind.

I want to share a bit of perspective that might help as you first years start the final three years of your fourteen years of medical training. No need to take notes, just going to share some old man experience. Whoever was on call last night, this may be a good time to catch up on much-needed sleep.

I don't know if you have noticed yet, but our patients give us a lot of gifts, sometimes out of appreciation, sometimes to curry favor, sometimes to deploy as a burnt offering to appease the cancer gods. We work hard for our patients, and like it or not, we think about them nearly twenty-four hours a day, seven days a week. They in turn are enormously grateful, so many of them express their gratitude with gifts—sometimes as simple as a thank-you card, sometimes a large donation to your research program. I have received more than thirty baseball caps logoed with the patient's favorite team or golf course. Over the years, we all amass a collection of various items given out of appreciation, maybe even love. Many of these objects remain quite dear, reminding us of a special patient or event. Next time you're in my office, take a tour of my "gift museum." I have a statue of a fiddler from Israel and a small copy of the Hippocratic Oath etched into a plastic replica of a stone tablet. I have a couple of painted rocks. As you might guess, I have a lot of poop-oriented gifts. Many of the items were obviously purchased in an airport gift shop or duty-free shop. For a while I got a lot of cologne, which made me wonder about my hygiene.

We also get a lot of food: cookies, doughnuts, cakes, exotic chocolate, not-so-exotic chocolate (both highly welcome), even the occasional samosa. For you new fellows, Christmas is amazing around a cancer center. So much food, so much chocolate. It takes us until Valentine's Day to get through it all, only to receive the next wave of treats—now all heart-shaped. Our favorite? Booze, of course. If you do your notes on time, I might be willing to share it with you!

Patients come to the clinic with a smile on their faces. I see a gift bag next to them, wondering if it's for the nurses, the staff, or better still, me. As I turn to leave, they stop me, and with a bit of pride, they offer the gift. I am secretly hoping for bourbon. Usually, I open it on the spot so the family can share in my joy—or explain the gift. But inside, not uncommonly, is a bottle, not of bourbon but of some obscure liqueur, a traditional drink from their home country that is reserved for special occasions. My family and I will love it! We hug, and I thank them. My oldest bottle is a red wine called Adria, jokingly given to all the graduating fellows by the infusion nurses in 1993. Adria is also the nickname of Adriamycin, "the red devil." Never opened, never will be. It means even more to me now that my wife has had six doses of Adria to treat her breast cancer. I love catching a young med student, nervously interviewing for a residency position, glancing over my head to see my collection of obscure booze nestled among many other gifts. The brave ones ask, but most don't. Maybe my eclectic museum improves our acceptance rate.

Just a reminder, the official policy is that we aren't really supposed to keep the gifts. As I recently was reminded, we work in the only service industry where co-pays but not tips are allowed. In China, the families of patients give the docs "red envelopes" full of money to ensure the best care—something maybe we should consider as part of healthcare reform? Still, given how genuine and deeply felt these expressions of thanks are, it would be rude not to accept.

My favorite piece of my office collection is a cloth wall hanging, hand-made by a former patient. On it are depictions of important places in my life: Duke, the University of Louisville, Georgetown, and even my church, all surrounding the outline of Kentucky, my birthplace. It could not be more thoughtful and impossible not to accept. Once a lovely patient of mine brought in a huge shopping bag containing a red, white, and blue crocheted blanket. Right on cue at the end of our visit, she withdrew it from the bag and kept unfolding it and unfolding it until at the end it was larger in area than the exam room we were in.

I looked at it in amazement and asked, "When on earth did you find time to make this?"

She smiled and replied, "Waiting for you."

She had spent most of her last months of life here in our clinic, and yet she channeled all that into a marvelous expression of love and gratitude.

Then there was another gift I received early in my career. I was covering for a breast cancer specialist who was out on maternity leave, so I saw her patients for a few months. The absolute worst part of an oncologist's job is giving bad news. On scan days, patients come to clinic anxious, hoping and praying that they are cured, that the scan is fine. As *we walk the halls, they try to catch our eyes and read our faces to get a sign, any sign, of how things are.*

In prepping for the next day's clinic, reviewing the patients' results I would be delivering, my colleague's patient had a "bad scan," and I was going to have to tell her the news. Before you go into a room with a bad scan result, you should always be prepared. First, you are likely to be in there for a long time, and your clinic will run late the rest of the day. Make sure you get the easy patients out of the way first; I will even take patients out of order if I know what's ahead. Once in the room, you have to know everything in the chart by heart without glancing at it even once so you can look the patient and family in the eye. You must have at least a proposed plan for the next steps. There is nothing worse than leaving a bad scan visit without a plan. Read your patient's reaction, and read the caregiver's reaction. Be prepared for hard questions. Be prepared to stop talking and wait for them to resurface. Answer questions kindly, gently, compassionately, optimistically, skillfully, but most important, honestly. You have just caused maybe the worst day ever for a family and friends; you have just set in motion a ripple that quickly grows into a shock wave. Everyone in the family soon will know what you just said—or at least their interpretation of what you just said. Remember, a surgeon's gift lies in the hands, an oncologist's in the spoken word. Both can hurt, but both can heal. Whatever you do, prep your clinic, know where the bad scans are, and be ready.

In this patient's case, her husband was with her. Gently but clearly I told her. She was not in any immediate trouble, but the scan was bad news. We were going to need to resume treatment for her cancer, and, no, it could not be cured. I answered all their questions. I offered to follow up if I learned more. We made plans to start the treatment, I ran our plans past her primary oncologist as promised, and we moved forward.

No tears, no obvious anger or distress. Just sadness, note-taking, and seeming acceptance.

Months went by, and it was Christmas. My friend was back from maternity leave, and I refocused only on my patients. 'Twas the season of giving, and we were all getting our usual cards, chocolates, and bottles. I came back to my office and found a lovely, beautifully wrapped gift on my desk with a card. I did not recognize the name right away, but then her face flashed into my memory. It was from the breast patient with the bad scan. I smiled, thinking how thoughtful. I opened it. Inside the shiny box was a small Christmas stocking. I looked inside and found a lump of coal.

I was only doing my job. I was the messenger. I did not make her cancer return. It was not my fault. But somehow, I always saw this lump of coal as blame, as anger, as pain that had to be shared, a reciprocal punch in the gut.

I keep this gift in my top drawer and see it almost every day. I pull it out to show our colleagues, when a young doctor is in my office feeling the stress of life, or a staff member is upset by being yelled at by some patient. I pull it out as a reminder of the pivotal, sometimes approaching godlike role we play in our patients' lives. I pull it out to remind us that we are far from godlike, and the impact of what we say and how we say it is unpredictable and unmeasurable. Our words become key chapters in our patient's family stories. Sometimes we are the heroes—the lovely wall hanging, the booze collection—and sometimes the villains. In case I ever need a reminder of where I can stand, I always have that lump of coal.

CHAPTER 17

Being Alone

I am terrible at being alone.

I am actually alone a lot, so I get plenty of practice—in my office, on a plane, in my car. But almost always I use the time to distract myself from the fact that I am alone. I work on a talk, finish e-mails, complete my charts, read nerdy stuff like grants, manuscripts, and new science research. When I am not actually doing something, my mind immediately goes on alert, wandering around looking for something to do. Fortunately, there is always my office to clean. If there is a stack of papers somewhere, if there is an old journal sitting around, if I have left "to do" notes to myself, I clean it all up before returning to my computer, to see if anyone has sent me something that needs urgent action, a big job, a small job, eager for anything.

I wonder how my patients are. I think about the ones who need a call to see how they are doing. I have a few minutes; maybe I can go up to the hospital wards and make an unexpected visit just to say hello. When all of that is done, I wander around the offices and check in with colleagues and our amazing staff. I ask how they are feeling and if there is anything I can do for them?

I text one of the kids: "What's up?" No immediate answer. Then they respond with the loving respect all parents of Millennials have grown to treasure: "quit using punctuation in texts it is annoying." (A text obviously in need of a semicolon, not to mention a capital Q.) Apparently they are not going to help break my boredom. I click around trying to come up with birthday or Christmas ideas for Liza. Sometimes inspiration comes, often not. I recheck my United Airlines app to see if I have made Global Services. Still no. I check to see who is pitching for the Nats tonight.

When bored at home, I watch bad TV. As with all aspects of our lives, Liza is a master at the TV. Not only does she know what to watch, she knows where to find it and how to record it. All the unlimited choices take investment, time commitment, attention, and ability I do not have. After having given up on my many requests to join her, she has left me behind. So now she watches all this culturally crucial stuff without me, and true to form, when she finds something truly great, she offers to watch it again—even the entire series of *The Americans*—this time with me. It took a global pandemic for me to finally accept her loving offer. Without Liza, I am watching a *Big Bang Theory* rerun. Without structure, a mission, or a purpose, when bored and idle, I make bad decisions.

Liza is my guide, my rock, my compass, and my moral rudder. She is my true love. I am neither exaggerating nor lying when I say that she was sent by God to rescue me. I had learned that I am no good on my own, no good without a map, a compass, or someone to show me true north. As long as she is with me, I would never be lost again.

Except inflammatory triple-negative breast cancer is almost always fatal. I was going to be alone again, rudderless, making bad decisions.

How would I go on? Would I remarry like my dad? What would the kids think of a new mother? No woman could ever live up to Liza. But I can't stand being alone. I have not been alone for my entire adult life. Maybe I could just date for a while. (Who would want to date me, forever in love with another woman?) How long does a grieving widower have to wait until he can date? Would our mutual friends keep me on the list? Would I continue to go to church? (Would I be able to believe anymore?) Would I continue to be motivated to work? Would I drink more? Would I travel alone? Maybe sell the house and get a fancy apartment downtown. Maybe move back to Lexington and be with my family.

I am a world-renowned oncologist, and my wife has the worst possible kind of breast cancer, and I don't even know how to work the fucking TV.

CHAPTER 18

The (Dis)comfort of the Chemo Routine

After Christmas, we all fell into our new schedule. Chemo every other Monday with all the attendant arrangements for everyone. My subsequent physical decline over the succeeding week, nausea the first few days, growing fatigue from day five on, and a slew of areas of physical discomfort that generally peaked on about days six and seven. A week after treatment, blood tests were ordered to monitor my blood counts as they might drop to dangerously low numbers. Then the second week my energy would improve, and my side effects diminish, until it was Monday morning, and the drill started all over again.

Without the support we received, I'm not sure we would have made it through as a family. In ways both good and bad, a routine masks the actual day-to-day effects of going through cancer treatment. There is a lot I don't remember about this period because of sheer monotony, and my guess is that the routine helped everyone get through, particularly Charlie and Emma. The change in my appearance over this period must have been disturbing to them, but when you are with someone all the time, the changes are less apparent. The baldness and wig were obvious, but the lost eyebrows and eyelashes were less so.

I actually learned to enjoy chemotherapy days. No one called, I didn't get e-mails on my phone in those days, and no one outside or inside the hospital bothered me. Lunch was provided, a snack room offered drinks and cookies, and all the people, even most of the patients, were funny and sweet. Claudine would come by for a chat. John would stick his head in to check on me and maybe eat some lunch. We spent a lot more time together during this period than we had in years—another benefit of my being treated at Georgetown. John could meet me at Dr. Liu's office for my pre-treatment visit and see me off to the infusion unit. Then he could go to work, stopping by if he had a few minutes or was on the unit anyway, and finally take me home at the end of the day. The fact that John was working removed a burden from both of us. He could take care of his wife while she got chemotherapy without having to take a day away from the office, and I didn't need to feel guilty about what he was not getting done.

Chemotherapy days had a unique feature, which I loved. The Lombardi Cancer Center had received funding for a program of arts and humanities for cancer patients, their caregivers, and the staff. Musicians, dancers, crafters, artists, and writers appeared periodically in the clinic and the infusion units. Sometimes someone played an instrument in the clinic waiting room. On several occasions, a dancer visited me while I was getting chemotherapy, and we did graceful exercises and movement, just the two of us. A writer from Ireland encouraged those of us getting treatment to write poetry. I made a lovely copper leaf pressed between two pieces of glass which still hangs in my kitchen. I came to call those Mondays "chemo camp."

The first day after chemotherapy, I always felt pretty good as I had spent the preceding day lying on the infusion center bed, napping and doing crosswords while the poison was dripped into me. In addition, I was on steroids to enhance the effects of the anti-nausea drugs. If you have ever taken steroids, you know they give you a lot of energy. That energy and the fact that I felt well meant that I kept up with my normal activities the first few days after treatment. I did have some side effects, and those put a crimp in my daily activities, particularly as the week went on.

Side effects. The term sounds so benign, like a slight rash or consti-pation. (Not that those are trivial problems. I have had them, and they are no fun.) But chemotherapy side effects are a nonstop onslaught of problems, and the longer you are on chemotherapy, the worse and longer lived the side effects are. I visited so many different doctors during this period for so many problems that cancer treatment became a full-time job. My admiration has no bounds for people who manage to keep working while undergoing chemotherapy.

Dr. Liu's written report after the first treatment was that I did pretty well. Some mouth discomfort, some mild nausea the first day, some fatigue on the third day. All in all, not bad. Dr. Liu prescribed some-thing called Magic Mouthwash to help with the mouth discomfort as that can cause people to cut back on their food intake. I had recom-mendations on what to avoid, such as spicy, sour, and acidic foods.

After the first treatment, I felt all right, pleased to have gotten through the intervening weeks before the second treatment without too much awareness of what the chemotherapy was doing to me, other than the many pills I had to ingest the first few days to keep side effects at bay. During the week after the second treatment, however, my side effects began to grow more severe. The first day after treatment, I woke up feeling fine, but as the day wore on, my stomach started to roil. I had a feeling at the back of my throat that seemed as if my esophagus was working overtime to keep the contents of my stomach where they belonged. I spent the day wavering between whether I should put something in my stomach or leave it empty as well as wondering if I could venture away from home in case matters worsened.

I made it through the day, but I still felt rather sick when Dr. Liu called the next day to check on me as she always did. "How are you feeling?" she asked. "Well, I am nauseated this time," I replied. "I haven't actually thrown up, but I feel more like I might." "Would you like more anti-nausea medicine?" I hesitated. Was it really that bad? Did I want to take another pill? Was I being a big baby? Being nauseated was part of the deal, wasn't it? I had been regaled by friends when I was first diagnosed of them holding back their mothers' hair while their mothers puked their guts into the toilet as a result of breast cancer treatment, and I didn't want that for me or any of my family. I also knew that those were stories of bygone years and that treatments and medicine for side effects were much improved. But it *would* be great not to feel nauseated at all, not to worry that I *was* going to throw up, either at home or somewhere else.

I was already taking a tried and true anti-emetic, Compazine, and steroids for the week after chemo, but they didn't do the trick. For the next cycle, Dr. Liu said she would add Emend, a newer and somewhat more effective anti-nausea drug. And a much more expensive one. Compazine was a couple of dollars per cycle of chemotherapy while Emend would set my insurance company back more than $600 per cycle. Dr. Liu didn't mention the expense, of course. Maybe she should have.

But John didn't hesitate when he called home later that day. I happily picked up the phone when I saw who it was. He asked how I was doing, and I casually responded, "OK. I'm still feeling a bit sick, and I told Minetta when she called, so she said she's going to add Emend next round." There was silence on the other end of the phone.

"Do you know how much that drug costs?" John asked with a real edge in his voice.

"Well, I don't like feeling sick," I shot back.

"The drugs you are already taking are fine. There's nothing wrong with a little nausea. You can still do things."

"But I don't like it, and I'm afraid it will get worse, and I *will* throw up. I need to do stuff!" I barked. I might have hung up on him at that point. He didn't call back. I was mad, and he was mad. This conversation wasn't going anywhere, and I didn't want to fight about it. It was my body, my nausea, my life, my decision.

And I'm embarrassed to say, I knew I wasn't going to pay any more for it.

Another one of John's favorite areas of pushback in the cancer world is the cost of cancer drugs. He frequently talked to me about new cancer drugs that might cost $25,000 a month, which added on average only two weeks to a patient's life. He makes that point in his lectures to other doctors as well, arguing that the cancer research community wasn't really trying to cure cancer, but only to extend life by a few weeks. There are not unlimited funds to pay for healthcare, he would say. Money was coming out of our pockets through Medicare or insurance, as few individuals pay out of pocket for their treatment. The downstream implication was that cuts have to be made elsewhere, or we all have to pay much higher premiums to cover the costs of these newer drugs. We all pay for them, he says, and as a society we should be sure that the cost to all of us is worth it. If we had to pay for these drugs ourselves, we would make a cost-benefit calculation, and that might lead to a different decision. I wholeheartedly had endorsed and in fact repeated what he preached.

Until my nausea increased. I hated how I felt and worried it would only get worse, so Dr. Liu offered a way out. This expensive drug was about me now and not some abstract cancer patient. When John quizzed me on how bad I really felt, I bristled at his attempt to quantify my discomfort. I had cancer, and I was enduring treatment that was pretty brutal. Wasn't that enough? Didn't I deserve to feel good? I didn't have any more time to give to cancer treatment than I was already. And yet I knew that John was disappointed in me, and I was disappointed in me as well.

I was a hypocrite. I should be practicing what he preaches and what I believe. If I had had to pay for the Emend myself, I wouldn't have taken it. The nausea wasn't more than that, and I'd rather have the extra money for fun or even un-fun but more important things. But in the health-care realm, someone else is paying, so we don't have to think about how much a medicine or treatment costs. When our insurance company won't provide something, we are incensed at its inhumanity. The trouble is that in a world of finite resources, "humanity" to one person or group of people may very well require "inhumanity" to others. John diplomatically backed down, and I cost my insurance company and its policyholders $600 per cycle to keep me feeling a little better.

The more I reflected on my situation, the more confused and overwhelmed I felt. There was too much information, most of it in a language I didn't really understand. I had no idea why I was on the trial I was on. At my visit with Dr. Liu before the third cycle, I asked her again what the rationale was behind a clinical trial of six doses of Adriamycin/Cytoxan and six doses of Taxol, as opposed to four and four, the standard-of-care treatment. She reminded me that a study had shown "a small but statistically significant survival benefit" for patients like me on "dose dense" chemotherapy, and so now this was the standard of care. The thinking behind the additional doses of these drugs in the trial was that six doses of each might provide more of a survival benefit than four.

Each session took a bit more out of me. Round one, a bit of nausea, an unavoidable nap on day three, mouth irritation starting on day six. Round two, increased nausea, smaller meals to quell the sensation, the need for more and better anti-emetics. I was more tired, and I had to take things a bit more slowly. I increased the number of times I gave in and lay on the sofa for a bit, during the week if I could and particularly on the weekend. It was partly because I did feel weaker on days five to eight of the cycle and partly because John was home. Having meals made for us was a huge help for the first few nights after chemotherapy, and I was able to put something together other nights, but I "flaked out" on the weekends when backup was on hand. Fortunately, John seemed happy to take over in the kitchen for dinner. I still handled the kids' breakfasts and lunches every day, or at least on the days they didn't buy lunch at school.

Each dose of chemotherapy brought with it more and more uncomfortable side effects. One day after round three of chemotherapy, I felt pain when I defecated, and I noticed some blood on the toilet paper when I wiped. I've had rectal tears before, so I wasn't too worried, but normally the bleeding and pain would stop after a few days, and this time they did not. Apparently, the chemo was drying my skin, and my rectum was no exception. The nausea continued, but it wasn't debilitating, thanks to the many medications I was receiving during and after chemotherapy. I needed to keep something on my stomach at all times the first few days after treatment, and rich, creamy foods were the best, so I added a daily hot chocolate mid-morning and a cream soup at lunchtime. I was having chemotherapy, so I figured I deserved some edible treats, too. I was surprised when I put weight on during chemo, but I don't know why. The short answer is that I was consuming more calories and exercising, even moving, less.

The Saturday morning after the third cycle of chemotherapy, I got out of bed and immediately felt sharp pain in my feet. I let out a small "ouch" as I stood up. John was quick to tell me that this was an expected side effect of the chemotherapy called hand-foot syndrome, or scientifically, "plantar erythrodysesthesia." It is caused by the chemotherapy affecting the growth of skin cells or small blood vessels in the feet and hands and damaging the tissues. Fortunately, I never had much pain in my hands, but when I put my shoes on, the pain in my feet increased. I felt as if I was walking on hot coals. The next day when I put heels on to go to church, I struggled to stand up in them. Walking from the car to church was agonizing, a reminder of what Jesus had suffered for me.

On Monday, I reported my symptoms to Dr. Liu because I wanted some relief before the following week when I would see her again. She recommended that I start taking NSAIDs (nonsteroidal anti-inflammatory drugs) for pain relief. She also recommended that I start using what turned out to be a wonderful cream called Bag Balm, a thick yellow gel consisting of an antiseptic in a petroleum jelly/lanolin base, which dairy farmers put on cow's udders to prevent cracking. It is disgusting to wear but has amazing results.

Despite the remedies, the pain in my feet worsened. By early February, I was crying and whimpering with each step to church on Sunday, even when I finally had the good sense to put on flat shoes. I called Dr. Liu again that Monday, and she asked me to come in on an emergency basis, as she could hear the distress in my voice. She originally had assessed my hand-foot syndrome at Grade 1, but that day she jumped it to a Grade 3. She had me increase my NSAID dose, which necessitated something for the heartburn that the additional NSAIDs might cause. My pill box overflowed.

We worked on the rectal pain, too, using stool softeners, Tuck's ointment, A&D ointment, and sitz baths. The pain and bleeding became such a problem, however, that I finally consulted my gastroenterologist, yet another doctor visit. He recommended Anusol suppositories during the first week after chemotherapy. However, I wouldn't use them during the second week, when my immune system would be at its lowest, because of the risk of introducing external bacteria into my body.

At my visit with Dr. Liu before my fifth cycle, the notes taken by John, my faithful scribe and caregiver, listed the following issues that had followed the fourth cycle: upper respiratory infection with tearing and a runny nose, sore mouth, chest pain, nausea, rectal bleeding, a rash, painful feet, and fatigue. "Painful feet" was an understatement. My feet hurt so much that I couldn't walk or even wear shoes some days. Dr. Liu decided that in light of how much pain I was in, we needed to reduce the dose of Adriamycin by 20 percent, and I should start taking vitamin B6 pills. For the fatigue, she added a drug called Aranesp to increase my red blood cell count, which would be administered intravenously when I was having chemotherapy. I also started saline drops and a saline nasal spray to help with the tearing and runny nose, additional side effects of the Cytoxan. Remember that under standard-of-care treatment for breast cancer, I would have been done with the Adriamycin and Cytoxan at this point.

Our good friend Claudine Isaacs told me later that she now uses my case as an example for her patients who ask for more chemotherapy, telling them that my experience seemed to demonstrate that there is a point past which the toxicities and therefore side effects of the chemotherapy drugs seem to multiply exponentially rather than in a linear way. Adding doses of chemotherapy does not seem to have a salutary effect, only a deleterious one. In the end, that seems to be what the clinical trial I was on concluded as well. If my discomfort helped in that conclusion, I am pleased to have spared other breast cancer patients from the level I endured after the fourth, and per the standard, normally the last cycle.

The reduction of the Adriamycin made a big difference in my feet. With some ibuprofen on board over the middle weekend, when the symptoms were the worst, I could wear shoes and walk again. My other problems all improved, too, with the administration of a pharmacopeia and anything CVS would sell me over-the-counter. Oncologists are amazing doctors. They not only have to know about a very complex disease but also have to be able to cope with every other part of the body because little seems to be spared the harsh effects of chemotherapy. Someone once described chemotherapy to us as spraying bug spray into your live insect collection to get rid of the bugs you don't want. Of course, you would never do that because you'd kill the bugs you wanted to keep. Nonetheless, that is how chemotherapy works.

Having an oncologist in my bed most nights while I was going through cancer treatment was both a terrifying and calming experience. Many patients agonize for hours and days about symptoms and side effects, wondering if they should call the doctor's office or night number, go to the emergency room, or do something else. I had seen John receive many a call from patients with just these questions. I could just ask my husband. He didn't always know the answer (Remember, he's a GI cancer expert, not a breast cancer expert), but he could give me some assurance that it could wait until daytime.

On the terrifying side, John wavered between panicked and blasé in his treatment of me. He seemed to worry about things that I thought were trivial, like the sore neck I had at the time I was diagnosed with breast cancer. The day we heard my diagnosis, when we got in the car to go to Georgetown for the MRI and CT scan, John looked at me somewhat forlornly and said, "You know, you've been having that neck pain...." I looked back at him, surprised at his concern. "That isn't cancer." I knew it wasn't; I don't know how. Maybe it felt more soft tissue than bone. Maybe I was delusional. I was certainly frightened, but not about that.

I also found his sudden concern with germs drastic. For Christmas, just after I was diagnosed, we had planned to visit John's family in Kentucky, but John angrily declared that he was not going to have me going to the bathroom at a truck stop while I was immunocompromised. He normally wasn't afraid of germs, even for his patients, and we were going to go in our own car and be with family, whose germs I had been exposed to for years. However, he insisted that we were not leaving Washington, apparently suddenly a city with no germs. When he got ideas in his head that seemed silly to me, they would make me anxious about symptoms about which I previously had felt fairly sanguine.

On the other hand, when he didn't seem concerned enough about things I thought were very important, my anxiety level didn't *decrease*, because I attributed his lack of concern to his traditional dismissal of my health problems as not serious. For instance, he dismissed the nausea, which dominated my thinking as I imagined four more cycles of chemotherapy, but I think he viewed it as inevitable for cancer patients and therefore not important. While I don't think he thought my being subjected to an extra two cycles each of both kinds of chemotherapy was insignificant, I'm not sure he really considered the short- or long-term consequences for me.

It's a tough road to walk, being an oncologist whose spouse has a cancer with a dire prognosis. It's also a tough road to walk, going through cancer treatment with a spouse who knows as much as the treating physician and far more than the patient.

CHAPTER 19

Never Go to Funerals

Rule one of maintaining your sanity and emotional stability as an oncologist: Never go to funerals. Funerals are for families and friends to celebrate the life of their loved one. They are command performances in order to gather and mourn the loss of a dear friend, spouse, parent, or increasingly frequent in my line of work, someone in the prime of life. Oncologists are neither members of the family nor friends of the departed who need time to stop and mourn the loss. Actually, on second thought, we are in need of such a time. But that does not mean I am going to do it at a funeral.

Obviously, I am no stranger to funerals, and some of them are actually almost enjoyable. If the dearly departed has lived a long and good life, left all business finished, organized the service hymns and readings, and died peacefully of a short, pain-free illness, then gathering to retell old stories, meet the extended family and friends, and hear surprising biographical details can fill your soul with warmth and joy at having known that person. It may even leave you feeling a bit closer to God. Sometimes, an unexpected bonus, the family has sprung for an open bar reception to follow. A lifetime's worth of favorite family pictures are on display. Jokes are told, and we catch up with old friends. We leave inspired by a life lived with decency and gusto, and we set out to be better people ourselves so we too can have a funeral like that one.

Most cancer deaths and funerals, aren't like this. Those who die of cancer are usually too young. They suffer terribly and lose their long battle too soon. Their bodies are beaten up, and their final selfies often capture hairless, emaciated outlines of their former selves. If the person was in the prime of life, or worse, pre-prime, then the turnout is standing room only. The only noise breaking the hush comes from the quiet management of flowing tears. Hugs leave soaked shoulders. At the reception, the conversation centers on how the survivors are going to manage. Do you think she will remarry? The oldest clearly would benefit from therapy. I guess the youngest will go back to college next semester. At least he is no longer in pain. Did you see the farewell video he shot for the children? She should have done one of those videos for the children. Who are all these people? The mood is dominated by a sense of unfairness and a fear it could happen to anyone. If indeed it did happen to us, could we fight, endure, and manage the fatal cancer diagnosis as well as our friend whom we now mourn?

Almost always, when a patient of mine dies, I call the surviving spouse or daughter. (It is never the son—sons are not classic caregivers and rarely are there when things get rough.) I express my sadness, my regrets about something we could have done better, and my reflections on the battle fought. I try to offer some advice to the family going forward and suggest that in a month or so, we might want to debrief together. I also offer one insight: The now-former caregiver will experience two losses. He or she will feel the obvious and expected absence of the person whom they did everything in their power to keep alive.

But because most surviving spouses have spent the last three to six months as a full-time caregiver, they suddenly just lost their full-time job. No notice, no farewell cake, no gold watch—just a lot of unfilled, empty time.

Flash back one to two years before. After a tap on the exam room door, I enter. "Hello, I am John Marshall," and a new doctor/patient relationship is about to start. When you first meet a new patient and his or her partner in life, friend, or family member, all conversation is directed almost exclusively to the patient. There are lots of eye-to-eye exchanges to feel each other out. The other person in the room is the observer and note taker, almost an intruder in this most intimate, intense discussion. The doctor doesn't really know anything about the other person in the room. Do the couple really like each other? Were they about to break up, but cancer got in the way?

Most caregivers appear at virtually every appointment. They are double-checking everything we do, keeping track of the treatment schedule, trying to keep life going along as normally as possible. Caregivers are critical members of the team, but those who insert themselves too strongly irritate us. Here are some of the classics: overbearing, guilt-ridden daughters; patriarchal husbands who know it all "because I read it on Facebook"; wives who assume "caregiver knows best" attitudes and whisper, "Can I speak to you for a minute outside the room without the patient knowing to tell you really what is going on?" I understand that their single-minded focus is on the patient. And that is the way it is…until the patient starts to die.

As a patient becomes weaker, unable to be the decision-maker, the conversation and decision-making naturally shift almost exclusively to the primary caregiver—even if the patient had mapped it all out for us.

Like the Constitution, the original document requires some interpretation for the current situation. What would they *really* have wanted?

By the time the patient dies, the caregiver and I usually have become quite close, confidantes in managing the end of life. We have talked privately about the impending realities. I have coached them through the rough times, reassured them that we really did do everything and that they really did look under every rock for a cure that was not there. I have given the caregiver permission to let go, to focus on comfort, to just be there.

This can be a tender period, at least when we all agree that it is time to move on. There is a true sense of release, peace, and comfort. A bond forms between us, sometimes one that endures and is rekindled every time I see them again. At the mall, at the 5K colon cancer run, at church, in the airport, caregivers from the past appear out of nowhere. We immediately recognize each other, sensing our common bond and our shared experiences, reminded of the sadness, the pain, and the loss.

Once the patient dies, the caregiver and I inevitably talk about the planned service, and while not explicitly stated, there is an expectation from the family that I will attend the service. At the very least, they would be honored if I attended.

There are so many reasons I do not go. First of all, professionally, I feel like a guilty failure. My inadequacies as his or her doctor are the reason why the patient died, right? If only I had done more, if only I had discovered the cure for cancer in time, everything would have been different. If only I had spent more time adjusting pain medicines or stopped by hospice to say good-bye, I could have made things smoother for the patient, the family, and the kids.

Second, if I do go, I will be introduced to the rest of the family as Joe's oncologist, and with each handshake, each tense hug, I again will feel like I have let these people down. When I have attended funerals, maybe because I knew the patient socially, the highly developed emotional barrier required to maintain the objectivity to be a good doctor, absolutely essential in the tool belt of every oncologist, crumbles. I am sucked into the sadness. The family remembrances are the hardest for me. I learn so much more about my patient's life, all the good the person did, all that will not get done. On the rare occasions I do attend, either because I was asked to be a part of the service or because I just felt obligated, I almost never leave feeling closer to God.

Third and maybe not immediately obvious—not exclusive to funerals nor as rare as you might think—some attendee, often an elderly family member or friend of the deceased, passes out. Others look around, hoping someone will come to the rescue. They remember they were just introduced to me as the amazing doctor (Did I mention my patient just died?) of the deceased and expect me to spring into action. We healthcare people make this social obligation look cool, but all doctors hate the "Is there a doctor in the house?" announcement. The worst is on a plane. Our initial reaction is to slump into our seat and hope that an ER doctor, or better yet an ICU nurse, gets there first. Oncologists are not known for their resuscitative skills. We know the basics. We are better at this than, say, a psychiatrist; we are better at this than almost any lawyer, but we still don't like doing it. By the way, if any airline executives are reading this, we enjoyed the free drink or extra miles you used to offer us for spending our flight in an airplane bathroom holding the head and checking the pulse of a vomiting tourist returning from Asia. Now we get nothing—no co-pay, no letter, not even a crummy bag of pretzels.

At Holly's funeral, a very old member of our nation's leadership was wheeled into the church. Secret Service agents stood watch. The church is a beautiful, classic colonial-style complete with boxed pews, each with a small swinging door guarding the entrance, adorned with its brass plaque with the name of some old slave-owning Virginia family claiming that spot for all eternity. This church is for those who like to kneel, so kneeling cushions are provided. As a low-church Protestant, I don't like kneeling; it hurts my bony knees. The elderly eminence was parked right in front of me and Claudine, who also attended the service. I was assigned to do a reading.

We watched as the venerable lawmaker was essentially lifted into the pew box, wheelchair parked to the side. Pillows repositioned, propped up, mostly he seemed aware of where he was. All I could think was that this guy was actually allowed to vote on stuff that mattered! After I returned to my pew from my reading, I watched him collapse, slumped over in his pew. There was a slight pause in the service, but as is common in formal church services, the show must go on. As quietly as we could and with help from staff and the Secret Service, Claudine and I extracted him from the box, moved him into the Fellowship Hall adjacent to the sanctuary, laid him flat on the ground, and assessed him. He had a pulse. He recovered with no specific intervention, just our kneeling over him and maybe our few unspoken prayers with curative powers. The Senate balance was at fifty/fifty at the time. Who knows where our country would be now if the outcome had been different. Talk about having the balance of power in your hands!

I was thirteen when I went to my first cancer funeral. It was for my mother. I still can't remember the last time I talked to her, the last words we said to each other, and the last time we hugged each other. In those days, children were not included in the details of death. My brother, sister, and I were protected.

Her funeral was quite a show. Calvary Baptist Church in Lexington, Kentucky, is a Baby-Boom-inspired Southern Baptist church. Made with red brick, white wood trim, and a towering steeple, the church holds hundreds, maybe a thousand when the balcony is full. The church was and still is a downtown fixture. A big choir is located behind the pulpit, and behind the choir, a curtain hides the tiled pool used for baptisms, the full-immersion style where my brother, sister, and I were all publicly dunked. This church was like a second home to me and was very important to my mom. The ministers, the adults, my Sunday school teachers, and my many friends were my extended family. It was here where I first learned about God, where I was first shoved in the back by God, and where I came to realize that God exists and has a hand in my life.

The church was packed. The single benefit about dying young is that the turnout for the funeral is amazing. Aunt Ann, my mother's sister, made us take pictures of everything and in every combination, posed around my mother's casket in front of the altar. I have no memory of the words said, just that we sat exposed in the front row. The only thing in view was my mother in the casket and the minister. Everyone else was behind us, hundreds of pairs of eyes staring at the backs of our heads. All our dearest friends and family were wondering to themselves how we were going to go on without her.

After the service, she was wheeled out and put in the hearse, and we all drove with our car lights on to the Frankfort Cemetery, about thirty miles away. It was actually quite a line of cars. Seeing all those people at the church and in the line of cars made me feel very proud and special. I knew my mother was a friend to many, loved by many, and mattered to many. This display of affection and support was one of the best moments of my life and somehow eased the pain of losing her then. The support and love by my friends and their parents carried me through my personal valley of the shadow of death. They really did not want to be there. They did it for us, for me. That is why you go to funerals, especially the hard ones.

If Liza had died of breast cancer, her funeral would have been like my mom's. I did not want that for me, for Charlie and Emma, her parents and sister, our friends, and mostly for Liza. When I first saw Liza's path report, I was sure she was going to die from the cancer. I knew what the odds were and what the road ahead looked like. I saw Liza looking like my curled-up, wispy-haired, eighty-pound mom. I saw our church, the one we were married in, the one where our children were baptized, the one where I have attended many funerals. Our church is a beautiful fixture in the heart of Georgetown. Inside, no pew boxes, no kneeling pads, no tiled pool, just words of Scripture on the walls. It is a place where I restore my regularly depleted soul. I imagined our church filled with our friends and family, standing room only, everyone devastated, everyone wondering how we would get on without her. There would be no jokes, no slaps on the back, no open bar. I would feel even lonelier and more lost than ever. I could see it all when I heard about her diagnosis. But I knew that I could not share my soul-deep terror with the one person on the planet with whom I share everything.

When a patient of mine dies, I hold my own, very brief, service. I pause, I look up, I smile, I ask forgiveness. Finally, I ask the patient's spirit to support me and join the chorus of angels I feel pushing me forward to find cures for cancer. The aim is to refresh me, to energize me to help the next person on their journey. Then I pick up the phone and call the surviving spouse, and I move on. But I never go to their funerals.

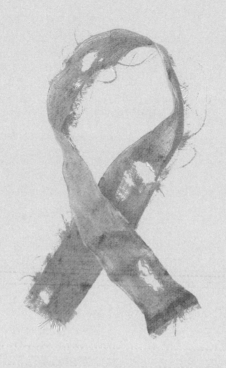

PART 5

What Are Oncologists Actually Thinking?

Simply by virtue of living with me, Liza already understood many lessons of a cancer diagnosis. She knew that life would never be the same. She knew that doctors don't know everything; there will be many uncertainties. Although this may have bugged her the most, I think she also knew that patients can never really understand all we tell them, no matter how hard they try. For some reason, there were several insights that most oncologists know, but that I could not share with Liza, at least not in the heat of the battle.

1. Maintaining hope is critical to obtaining the best outcomes.

A cancer diagnosis forces us to face our mortality. It forces us to acknowledge that our death may not be in some remote, do-not-have-to-face-now moment but much sooner than planned. Hope, the motivation that propels us to go on living, sustains us even through the darkest valleys of our lives. For each person facing a cancer diagnosis, there is a fine balance between incorporating a full understanding of mortality and maintaining hope for the future.

As members of a surprisingly small subset of doctors who deal directly with the topic of death, oncologists serve as escorts for patients and their families as they navigate the valley ahead. We must understand what it is that sustains our patients and their caregivers, then use that energy and focus in our treatment strategy. Without hope, patients become depressed and withdrawn, and some simply stop living. A key part of our job is to support them, to encourage them, and to make their life as positive as we are able.

Instead of focusing on death, we focus on life. We talk about cheating death, never tracking how many of the nine lives are left, always looking for a new treatment, trying to keep them alive—waiting on the next discovery, partly in the name of maintaining hope. We don't lie, and we try not to mislead. We see no need to pound the message of death into those patients who already "get it." There is actual medical literature showing that those with a positive outlook live longer, so let's make sure we keep all eyes looking ahead, full of hope.

2. Oncologists spin the message depending on the audience.

We are criticized by our non-oncology colleagues who think that we should be blunt, shoot straight, make it crystal clear to the patient with lines like "This cancer is going to kill you, likely in just a year or two, so get your affairs in order." Maybe for the right reasons, maybe because I hate to see the pain and shock and despair on my patient's face, I try to deliver a message of certain death from cancer that lands a bit softer. My colleagues would call it my coward's way of saying that someone is incurable.

For instance, a favorite line utilizes a bit of transitive logic: "Stage 4 colon cancer can be cured only by removing all the cancer surgically, and I think that you have too many spots of cancer for surgery to be possible." The patient is left to finish the equation. Another useful strategy is to refer to cancer in the third person. Pancreatic cancer, nearly always fatal, becomes "a demon of a cancer, and try as we might, we have not solved its mysteries." Often, we buttress a bad message with the hope for future discoveries. "There have been a lot of advances in cancer," I explain, "and while we have made progress in treating stomach cancers, we have not figured out how to cure yours. But hopefully with more time...."

We keep the flame of hope alive, hope being critical to maintaining quasi-normal daily living, the energy to move forward, and the sanity to stay strong.

3. Quality of life matters only if you are alive.

How much would you pay, and what would you sacrifice for a few extra months of life? In the abstract, when you are in perfect health, most of us casually wave off a few extra months as not worth suffering for. But when a loaded gun is pointed right between your eyes, you cannot help but try to get out of the way of the bullet. Most of my patients are facing a significantly shortened life, many fewer days than they had planned, and they need to start considering what they will give up to live a few more. To introduce this previously unconsidered yet critically important element of their future decision-making, I ask two questions that I only became brave enough to utter after my experience with Liza and her cancer. First, I ask, "What do you do for fun?" I ask this as an icebreaker to understand patients' priorities, hobbies, and joys. What I listen for in their responses are the things that they eventually will have to give up, goals they will not reach, and sacrifices they will have to consider.

The second is less subtle, and I save it for the end of our visit: "So how long do you want to live, anyway?" After looking a bit taken aback from my question, most respond with the ever-hopeful target of "at least eighty-five to ninety years old." We exchange brief agreeing smiles, and then I redirect us to reality, adding some major trade-offs, many that they don't know now, but they probably will face in the near future. "What if you couldn't drive?" I ask. "What if you were too tired to go out, too tired to travel? What if you were totally dependent on others? What if you were in terrible pain?"

Almost immediately the priorities shift. The patients' wheels turn as they calculate the algorithm of loss and the worth of time. Their answers generally follow these general themes: "I want to be comfortable. I don't want to live like that, all suffering, no joy. I don't want to burden my family."

They now can envision a point ahead when, even though that gun is still pointed at them, time is no longer what's most important, and quality of life becomes the primary driver. One of the major criticisms levied at my specialty is that we wait too long to engage our patients in quality-of-life discussions, typically reserved for too close to end-of-life, often deployed as we try to dissuade our patients from trying one more "Hail Mary" treatment. Frankly, if we followed our colleagues' advice and brought inevitable death up earlier, we would risk losing that precious commodity of hope. (See #1 above.) We know our timing is bad when, as soon as we begin the quality-of-life discussion, the patients' faces immediately sour, and their bodies physically recoil, ducking out of the loaded gun's path and clearly signaling that it is time to change the subject, doc.

After Liza's cancer, I have found it easier to think about quality and quantity as two bank accounts, both with some startup funds deposited in them. If a treatment works, you can add some cash to the quantity account (increased survival), but you will need to withdraw some from the quality account to pay for it (side effects). The exact amount of each investment and the eventual return is hard for us to predict. For example, some treatments simply do not work, costing a great deal in side effects, draining the quality account, and adding nothing to quantity. At their worst, the side effects can be bad enough to take a few bucks away from the quantity account, unexpectedly losing precious time. Some patients are willing to risk a big stack of their quality bucks, gambling that the investment will pay off in quantity. Others are more conservative, unwilling to risk major side effects for unknown improvements in survival. And in some cases, it falls to us doctors to take a reading of both accounts and advise patients as to their best investment strategy. Can a patient tolerate (afford) the risks, and for what gain? At some point in our journey together, taking a fresh look at the accounts, we come to a time when there is not enough left in the quality account to justify the possible bump in quantity. It's time to stop treatment, time to retire and use what you have saved in the two accounts to live out your days.

4. Putting more chips on the table does not guarantee a win.
Patients in Liza's situation face a different value system from those with incurable cancers. Liza did not face certain death. She may have been cured by the surgery alone, but were we willing to bet on that? Liza's calculation was much clearer than quality vs quantity; it was life or death. Her odds of being cured by surgery alone were roughly 40 percent—far from a sure bet. To increase the chances of a cure after surgery, we give systemically administered treatment. We call this post-operative "adjuvant therapy." The treatment may be thought of as adding a few more chips to the table, increasing the odds of a win. Oncologists have a bad case of "regret avoidance." Adjuvant therapy—chemo either before or after surgery to clean up any wandering cells—is our big chance for maximum impact. Don't back down; don't be too nice; this is our chance to CURE this patient. They can take it. No regret. (Plus, this is a different kind of ounce of prevention because we could be sued by some bottom-dwelling lawyer for our failure to be sufficiently "dose intense.")

If we really believe that more is better, then how much chemo can we give? What is the ceiling? Is there a limit? If you have given the limit, we did all we could do. And yet there are still those lingering, inconvenient uncertainties: Are we really sure that more is better? Are we sure that the subsequent damage justifies the increased treatment?

It is only recently that we have started to question the physical, psychological, and cognitive impact of our aggressive treatment approach on our patients. We are increasingly recognizing that our zeal to give the most intense treatment possible may have cured a couple more people than our old standard of care, but at a cost of so many more people left with a lifetime's worth of physical reminders and true disabilities. Some may be "mild," a bit of neuropathy, bone marrow that's slightly beat up, or early menopause. Some may be quite serious, like a second cancer, debilitating fatigue, uncontrollable bowels, inability to eat a normal meal, and chronic pain. Isn't it better to be alive with new problems than to be dead? Breast cancer researchers have spent decades pushing the envelope of dose intensity. Higher doses, more doses, pushing to the edge and back—repeat times four, times six, will anyone give me eight cycles?

In an infamous set of trials, the breast cancer community pushed the envelope too far: Researchers performed a series of trials using high-dose chemo rescued by bone marrow transplants as adjuvant therapy for moderate to high-risk breast cancer. Bone marrow transplants are treatments that take patients beyond the edge—after totally wiping out patients' bone marrow with extremely high doses of chemo, then rescuing patients by giving them their own previously harvested and stored blood cells. When I started at Georgetown, I cared for patients in these trials. We exposed many women—some of whom might have been cured already—to this extremely intensive treatment.

As it turned out, bone marrow transplant treatments were an insurance policy that proved fatal, offering no additional benefit. In the 1990s, this was the state of the art, or at least what we were all sure was going to be the state of the art. The problem was that there was little to no evidence that this was a good idea. The trials we were doing were based on prior results that we later found out had been intentionally falsified. We were escalating the risk to our limits, pushing hard in a direction that was supported by fraudulent results, that had no added value. Thinking back, Liza would have been eligible for these trials.

When I was on call one weekend doing rounds, I went to see one of my colleague's patients. She was about fifty, with her husband at her side. She had been diagnosed with breast cancer, and her surgery done a few months before might already have cured her. Standard chemo that she had completed might have added to her chances of cure, but she was at moderate to high risk of still having cancer cells somewhere. She wanted to do anything she could do to be cured and live a normal length of life, no matter the risk, just like Liza. She wanted no regret, just like Liza. She enrolled in the bone marrow transplant trial.

Sitting vigil in the ICU on this particular Saturday, neither the patient nor her husband remembered the enthusiasm they felt the day they signed up for the trial. She had no blood cells, the rescue of her bone marrow failed, and she was falling into the abyss and would not return. They did not remember the many serious warnings that were spelled out during the informed consent process. All they remembered was that this was going to increase the chance for a cure and the hope in their minds that translated into a promise.

They decided that they needed to take their anger out on me. I was not their doctor, only the weekend-covering junior guy. I simply listened and took the blows for the team. I expressed my apologies, my sorrow, my attempts at understanding. Once released, I too was angry—at our world, our ignorance, our crazed enthusiasm for dose-escalating, envelope-pushing treatments. Angry at the breast cancer juggernaut, which should have known better. She died two days later. If she had not participated in the clinical trial and opted for the current standard of care, she probably would still be alive. I hoped that at least the bone marrow transplant trial she was on was going to produce progress. As we now know, it did not.

So now, this is where we were with Liza: The surgery covered 40 percent, and her chemo added 20 percent more, but at a cost. There was nothing that we knew about at the time that could cover the remaining 40 percent. How many chips do you want to buy? Place your bets, and let's spin the wheel!

Oncologists are not typically big gamblers, at least not at casinos. Our gambling tables are in clinic, and we work for the house. We explain the rules of the game. We know the odds. We can estimate the cost of the chips and the likely chances of winning. We try to assess our patients' interest in taking risks, guiding them on where to place their bets. It's always easier when it is not your money. It is only one spin, one roll of the dice; no second chances. The patient wins or loses on the one bet. We celebrate when they win; we are there to console when they lose.

In placing an educated bet on adjuvant chemotherapy, a patient has no way of truly understanding the real cost of a chip. All the information is in a new, foreign language; facts are vague, and details are unquantified. Not to mention, the entire situation is very scary. When faced with win or lose, life or death, of course we put as many extra chips on the table as we possibly can, even if the improvement in odds provided by one extra chip is small, even as low as 1 percent.

You would be surprised at how few patients actually want to know the details of the game they are about to play. Most patients don't ask directly for their odds if they do nothing more, or the odds that more treatment will help and by how much. More often they step up to the table, put down their chips wherever we tell them to, blow on the dice for good luck, and let them fly.

5. Statistically positive results do not always translate into something that is clinically meaningful.

There is no question that we are making progress in the war on cancer, but much of the progress is coming in very small steps. Let's say I offer you two options, treatment OLD or NEW. Treatment NEW involves a new medicine, a bit more toxic than OLD, but was found to give better results than OLD by a small but statistically significant amount in a large trial that just was published in the *New England Journal of Medicine*. You probably would take NEW. You would want the best that cancer research has to offer. If instead, I tell you that there is a new treatment that is more toxic and more expensive and actually fails to add any benefit above the standard-of-care treatment 97 percent of the time, you would take OLD. Watch out for our sales pitch—it can be deceptive. We can make 3 percent look worth it or alternatively absurd depending on which sales pitch we use. Not all progress is worth the cost.

6. Most clinical trials are negative.

Clinical trials are my life, my scientific raison d'être.

Drafting patients to enroll in trials is a core mission in my life. I am proud of our research successes. I just want more, and I want us to be smarter about it. We continue to value small gains, and in order to detect those, we must do big trials. A large group, often thousands of patients, is randomized to receive either the standard of care or the standard of care plus something. The "plus something" treatment we hypothesize will result in more cures, the trial designed to find a delta as small as 3 percent, a detail we almost never tell patients, and they never ask.

I am in the business of designing, running, interpreting, and sharing the results of clinical trials. It's one of the most important reasons that I work at a cancer center. The volunteer patients are the risk takers, the true soldiers in the war on cancer. They see the current standard as unacceptable or at least sub-optimal. They too want to make progress, to help move the bar, and to leave the world a better place. They are willing to lead the charge, to climb out of the trench into incoming gunfire, even if victory means at best moving the bar by 3 percent.

It is also true, however, that trial participation is also my *"raison de promotion."* While not directly incentivized for enrolling a patient on a trial, I am judged for this, and it factors into academic promotions. In order for a cancer center in the United States to be designated as an NCI Comprehensive Cancer Center, a badge we wear proudly and work hard to maintain, we must enroll a certain percentage of our patients in trials. Translated, this means I have to have patients who agree to participate, or we could lose the coveted NCI status. To maintain my objectivity and remove as much conflict of interest as possible, I never open a trial or offer a trial to a patient in which I myself would not enroll.

This government standard applies to every NCI center, an employment expectation for every clinical researcher. We track our accrual to trials closely. If we fall behind, we are coached to step it up a bit. Over the years I have been the head coach, the associate director for clinical research, and that was my position in 2006, when Liza was diagnosed.

I found myself in a funny position. I was responsible for our center's clinical research output. That meant I got career credits for each one of the three trials my wife enrolled in. Wasn't this the ultimate conflict of interest? I know that she didn't just do that for me, as we had discussed clinical research often, both of us expressing our belief that participation is almost our duty. I am not sure if she found comfort in participation, but I know I did.

7. I was glad all of this was her choice and not mine.

CHAPTER 20

Going Public

A few weeks after Liza started her chemo, still feeling numb but knowing that the show must go on, I was on the road to speak at a meeting in Florida. As part of the meeting, I was interviewed by Neil Love, a breast oncologist who remains world renowned for his educational programming. In those days, Neil recorded interviews with cancer specialists using high-tech boom microphones hanging over their heads as he picked the experts' brains on the latest data and the immediate implications in day-to-day practice. The recordings were cleaned up, burned onto a CD, and mailed to everyone in our field. It was how we all kept up before the more modern websites and Twitter. The CDs were played back during commutes to and from work. Listening to Neil Love interviews was the way we all learned, and being interviewed by Neil Love was and still is an honor. It was a sign you had made it. At last, I was playing Broadway.

My lecture style is relatable, homey, the Kentucky boy in the big city. I use stories to teach, and they reappear over and over again, as anyone who works with me or lives with me will tell you. (If it worked once, it will work again!) Often my stories are from my past, or about my kids and Liza, and I never asked their permission before I publicly outed them. It's not as if I follow a script. I just have found that family stories are a great teaching device, keeping the audience's attention while sharing my personal bits with those in the room. Maybe this is a way for me to be close to the kids even when I am far away.

In Emma's middle school years and before she matured into an obsessively organized person, her room was a mess, true entropy at work. She did not want us to touch any of it. To her, it had order; it was not her fault that we did not understand its subtle structure and purpose. Emma's room became the perfect model to explain the randomness of cancer. One look at her room mirrored the seemingly endless randomness that I was trying to comprehend, measure, and restore back to non-lethal order. I shared with many audiences large and small, live and on video, that Emma actually understood her self-generated disorder, and we should respect her wish for it to remain as it lies. We simpletons could not see the downstream impact and the connections among her seemingly random placement of items—if we picked up one of her socks, then of course she would not be able to find her math book. While the story always got a laugh, it also made the point of our mission as cancer researchers. And it made Emma's room and her brief period of messiness known to many around the world. Without their informed consent, my family was out there, part of my act. We were the cancer family, and I shared even the most intimate family details if I thought it could help make progress in our war on cancer.

I was on the road again just as Liza was starting her chemo. I was going to be gone only one night. I was sure that Liza could handle everything at home without me. I could not turn down the invite to the meeting or the chance to be interviewed by Neil Love.

I sat down across the table from Neil, with the almost comically furry boom mics, one in front of each of us, blocking us from seeing face-to-face. As an innocent icebreaker, he asked me how I was, and for the first time since Liza's diagnosis, I shared my thoughts and feelings.

Neil started off, "You mentioned a couple of times you've alluded to your personal experience. Do you want to talk about it?"

"Um, I don't know if it's useful to you."

"I think it would be."

I love an audience, "I don't think Liza will mind. So after all the years that I have been publicly jealous and bad-mouthing breast cancer, it pays me back by visiting my house—my wife was recently diagnosed with Stage 3 breast cancer. We've gotten to experience all the things we talk about: the fear, the decision-making around treatments, the management of side effects. She had mucositis; she's lost her hair, and she looks very cute, but she's lost her hair."

"And I have to tell you, it's made me a born-again symptom management guy. That even a little bit of mucositis that my wife had on cycle one was enough for her to do all the things she could do to try and prevent it. I would have, two months ago, said to my patients, 'A little bit of mouth sores? Didn't prevent you from eating much? You're good. No need to change doses.' But it's really changed me in that way. I am all over even the smallest side effects now."

Neil kept going, now asking about the kids.

"How have your children gotten involved with this? What have you been saying to your children? What's happening?"

"Well, our kids are a little odd in the fact, you know, as any oncologist's kids would, they know what's going on. I mean, my kids have gone on rounds. They know what cancer can do and what it looks like."

"How old are they?"

"Ten and fourteen. So they're pretty savvy about the whole thing, and I've been so pleased with them. On the one hand, they've sort of recognized what we're all going through, but on the other hand, they're still bad children, so that means everything's normal. I mean, their rooms are still messy, and they still need fussing after, so they're not walking around on eggshells. We're pretty open about everything. They know what's going on, not gory details, but they know what's going on, and they're going on with their lives, and that's what we want, frankly. So pretty well-informed kids. We're lucky."

I told him everything, and I had a lot to say.

"What's been going on between you and your wife emotionally," Neil asked, "in your relationship?"

With a laugh, I responded, "We like each other more—this has really turned into a therapy session. Actually, in many ways, it's been quite good. We were both very busy people. You know how busy we are, as docs on the road and clinic and all of that. She's been very involved in my kids' school, on the board of my kids' school. She and I teach Sunday school every Sunday morning. You know, there's a lot of stuff that we're involved with our kids and in life and in the community."

I continued, "So in a sense for ourselves, we were running in two very busy, parallel paths, taking care of our kids and loving each other. We both think we're changing the world, and we're there supporting each other as we do it, so there wasn't any marital problem or anything. You know, we've been married a long time, but it's pushed us back together. Her breast cancer is a joint activity, so it's allowed me to refocus on what's important at home, too."

Neil drilled down a bit deeper, "Can you talk a little bit about how this experience has changed your perspective and your wife's perspective?"

"I think we were pretty much trying to live every day as we could. I mean, being a cancer doctor makes you appreciate every day. It really does. So it's made me impatient to be a better doctor, to be a better dad, to be all the things that you want to be, because you never know when the rug gets pulled out. The number of people who have come to our aid, I mean our freezer's full; I get rides for the kids anywhere. The people from work, the people from church, the people from school who come out to help you. The old 'It takes a village.' Well, it takes a village to, you know, get through something like this.

"And as oncologists, we're only seeing the two people who show up in the exam room. And what we don't realize is the pyramid of infrastructure that it took to get that patient through that cycle and get them into the next cycle and get them delivered on time with counts and all of that. We don't understand the ripple effect of telling people bad news."

At this point, I was on a roll. I somehow didn't realize how much I had to say, how much had been pent up inside me since Liza had gotten her diagnosis. Sitting in that quiet room, with the furry mic hanging there, talking to another doctor as empathetic and well-informed and curious as Neil was cathartic. I couldn't have stopped if someone had shoved a sock in my mouth.

"I'm pretty good at telling people bad news," I said. "We all are as oncologists. It's sort of a trait we share. But if we felt the ripple of every piece of bad news we gave and took it home, we'd go crazy. Particularly right after my wife's diagnosis, every time one of my patients had a bad CT or every time the biopsy was positive, I was feeling the ripple. And it was really a striking thing for me.... So I'm telling Mrs. Jones that she's got something going on, and I see in her eyes what I felt in my own heart, just a week or two earlier. And before, that was less powerful for me. I knew what I was doing, but I didn't feel the magnitude of what my patient's dinner table discussion was going to be like that night. So having lived it once, it's really sharpened that feeling. And I hope...I can't maintain that sort of intimacy, you know, twenty times a day, but hopefully it will make me even better at being sensitive to, making sure they get all the information they need...for that dinner table conversation."

"Do you think this is going to make you more effective as a physician?"

I didn't have to think long to answer that question because it was one that I had been preoccupied with since Liza's diagnosis. "I didn't know at first. So far I think so. My clinic slowed down. I'm taking more time. And I didn't know if I was going to have to get away from the clinic. And, actually, right now I'm quite drawn to it and the chance to make that patient's experience as good as we can make it through a rough time."

"So you're more aware of your importance?"

"Yeah, absolutely. You know, having hung on the words of, frankly, one of my colleagues as they talk about side effects and treatment and the like, you realize just how important those words are."

Neil added, "And there's a fundamental issue about how close we can get to our patients and not lose our minds, so to speak."

I knew exactly what he meant. "I think it's a necessary thing. I really do. I think there has to be some distance. As an example, we had a choice between very good breast physicians at my hospital, at Georgetown Lombardi, one of whom happens to be one of my best friends. Our families go out and do things, so of course, we immediately went to her. But then we realized that she couldn't really be the objective physician we need."

"It's one of the challenges, and we've talked about this before in colon cancer. Before, our patients typically died so fast we never got to know them well. Now as our treatments have improved, we're getting to know them. We get to know their kids. We know them for two, three, four years, and we know we're going to watch them die. And frankly, while I love that they are living longer, when they die, it's a lot harder than it used to be."

I had lost track of time. When I paused and looked at my watch, nearly an hour had passed. When Neil had run out of questions, he looked around the mics at me. The mics had served as something analogous to a psychiatrist's couch, imposing liberating Freudian distance that allowed my clearly therapeutic reflections to come so freely.

Neil had thought that the recording could be of interest to our field. But this time, of course, I would need family pre-approval. That evening, I called Liza and shared the details of the experience. Liza is not so public; she is practical. "Let's listen to it, and then we will see." A few weeks later, we received an edited version. She and I listened to it on our own, without the other. We also shared it with the kids. Without much concern or fanfare, all three gave their approval for my interview to go public.

This level of public exposure was different, so much more personal than a cute story to jazz up a lecture. This was giving a large audience an inside look into our personal experience, a kind of early reality TV. I had cultivated a reputation as someone who slammed the breast cancer industrial complex, and now the breast cancer industrial complex critic's wife has breast cancer. Let's listen in.

And listen in they did.

It felt as though everyone in the oncology community, coast to coast, listened. Maybe there was some mocking retribution for taunting the breast cancer gods. Mostly I received a flood of e-mailed expressions of concern and support. Many shared that they found the interview helpful and that they had better insight into their patients as a result. These people knew how bad Liza's cancer was; they understood the probabilities. They worried about us. They wanted a follow-up. Did she die? How is he dealing with that? Almost everywhere I went, someone would walk up to me and ask, "How's your wife?" Not in the cheerful, collegial, small talk, normal way. Now *I* got "the mournful oncologist looks."

While going public with our story may not have cured Liza, it certainly had a dramatic impact on her care. One of the expressions-of-concern e-mails I received was from my former boss, Marc Lippman. Marc is one of the world's experts in breast cancer, incredibly smart, and a great guy to have on your team. He is always on the cutting edge of breast cancer research, but brutally blunt, often for effect. One time on a nationally televised interview, he actually said that we could dramatically reduce breast cancer in the world simply by castrating all the thirteen-year-old girls—removing the ovaries of every thirteen-year-old girl. No ovaries, no estrogen, no breast cancer. We all waited for the "Of course, there is no way we would do that" follow-up, but it never came—just a cold piercing stare into the camera. Clearly influencing my own style, I always appreciated his boldness, his willingness to speak the truth even if only to shock and to refocus our path forward.

When Liza was diagnosed, Marc had left Georgetown, taking his eminence in the breast cancer field to the University of Michigan in Ann Arbor. I had not heard anything from him for several years, so the appearance of his name in my inbox was a bit odd. We were a few months into Liza's treatment. Many had reached out as they heard about Liza, but Marc would not be one to send a Hallmark message of support. I opened the e-mail. In all lowercase, e.e. cummings–like, the e-mail said:

"your wife needs a platinum, Marc."

Platinums are a class of chemo drugs that are in fact derivatives of the heavy metal found in many fancier pieces of jewelry. Here were drugs I was familiar with and an expert in how they work and managing their side effects. They are given intravenously. They are rough drugs, causing nausea, fatigue, neuropathy, hearing loss, vision changes, kidney damage, hair loss, low blood counts, and much more. To give cisplatin, the original of the class, we have to give at least a liter of normal saline before and after. We give the drug with a diuretic just so it doesn't knock out the kidneys as the drug passes through them. Before some of our newer anti-nausea drugs were invented, we had to admit patients to the hospital for strong sedation so they would not remember the brutal nausea it caused. Carboplatin, the newer cousin, is so toxic to the bone marrow that we have to calculate a precise dose each time we give it based on the patient's kidney function. As a class, they transformed the treatment of testicular cancers and are widely used in many cancer types, but there was no evidence at all that they worked in breast cancer. What the hell was Marc talking about?

In the interview, Neil Love had asked, "You mentioned that the decision was made to enter a clinical trial, and you mentioned that it was the SWOG study that's looking at two different forms of, sort of, dose-dense, metronomic, AC, Taxol, growth factors, you know, major therapy here. What led you to enter that study, you and your wife?"

When I answered, I described my commitment to clinical trials. "I'm a major advocate for clinical research, and so the trial was presented to us, and I think my wife threw that bone to me.... She has a relatively aggressive tumor. And so the idea of having extra chemotherapy, said from the guy who wasn't going to get a drop of it, seemed like a good idea. Each of the arms seemed OK to me. So for all of those reasons, not knowing what was the right thing to do, feeling that we needed to do more than just regular dose-dense because we were scared. You know, a tumor that grew up overnight with positive nodes. She had a mammogram three months before that was negative. So there was the fear factor of wanting to do more, being more aggressive than standard. For all of those reasons, that trial attracted me.

I continued, "I have to say, after the second cycle of AC, my wife looked at me and said, 'And I've got to do four more of these? Why?' She meant instead of two more, which was standard. So our fear has diminished now, and hopefully it's going to stay down, but we've kind of settled in now that we're doing something about it and just getting through it."

Marc's e-mail came right as Liza was getting her sixth cycle of AC.

Liza was bald, beat up, determined. Triple-negative breast cancer was a relatively new thing back then—considered worse than other kinds, more likely to spread, less responsive to the existing therapies. No magic bullets for this one yet. But researchers were learning and learning quickly. Platinums were just beginning to show promise as a potential magic bullet for her cancer.

As I looked at his e-mail, my mind began to race through all the algorithms involved in this decision. A platinum drug was not a part of the trial. There was only early evidence that treating Liza with this would help. If we took Marc's advice, Liza would have to come off the trial, and given my own history of annoyance when one of my patients withdraws from a trial, I felt guilty even considering it. Withdrawing would mean that the research team had essentially wasted their valuable time on us. Liza had signed a document committing to seeing this through. If she withdrew, she would not contribute to the breast cancer research machine all we had promised. Liza would become an asterisk in the publication, skewing the results. Minetta, a traditionalist and not one to make a move like this lightly, would have to agree with a plan that would mean even more chemo, more even than the extra amount Liza already had received on the trial. It would mean more side effects, more intense nausea, a higher risk of neuropathy.

But platinum could be the magic bullet.

We didn't have much time to decide given the implications of taking this step. We talked to Minetta, Claudine, and other breast experts. We got a lot of "I don't knows" and a few "might be a good idea but no firm evidence." Then there were the cautionary statements of how it "will not be easy at this point, given all the chemo she has already had." All I could think about was that some of these people had once said that bone marrow transplants were the magic bullet for breast cancer. Years later, and after many women were harmed, they discovered that was totally wrong. How could we trust them on this idea about platinum?

We were surrounded by excellent, contradictory advice—advice we had not asked for directly, advice that was provided as a side effect of going public. That meant, in the end, it was up to us. It was our decision.

We oncologists drop the "it is your decision" burden on our patients all the time. We find ourselves in unknown waters with unproven therapies—maybe someone, somewhere, has published an abstract suggesting it might help. We want to consider a new option, particularly if a patient is interested. We are really good at describing the pros and cons of what we know to try to paint the picture for the patient as clearly as we can. We then document in our chart (to protect ourselves from lurking lawyers) that we aren't entirely sure what the hell we are doing, that we described everything to the patient, and in the end, the patient wanted the treatment. They chose it, no longer my fault, no longer my responsibility. If they survive, we claim a victory. If they are harmed, or worse still, if they die, it was not our fault; we only did what they wanted us to do.

Liza and I talked a lot about this. Neither of us wanted to be branded as clinical trial quitters. Neither of us wanted more chemo. Neither of us wanted Liza to die. She could take it; we could get through this either way, and we could justify either path. In the end, we concluded that it was better to intensify the battle even if Liza was left more injured, even for unknown added benefit, than to lose. We added the platinum.

Even though I am sure the chart says this was all our choice, it was not our idea—I did NO research into Liza's cancer. I never called Marc to discuss his suggestion. I replied to his e-mail with an equally brief "Thanks." He had heard about Liza's illness only by my going public to the entire cancer community, my big mouth, feeding my ego. This had better work.

CHAPTER 21

Platinum, But Not the Pretty Kind

On February 26, 2007, I finally finished with the first half of my chemotherapy treatment, having received my last cycle of Cytoxan and Adriamycin. I felt like crap. It was not as crappy as I had felt after the fourth cycle, thanks to the decrease in the dosage of Adriamycin and a boatload of medications to remedy the multitude of pains in various parts of my body, but everything seemed exhausting. I had to piece myself together in the morning just to look normal: Insert the prosthesis in my bra, put on the tinted makeup to cover the pallor of my skin, pencil in my missing eyebrows, tug the scratchy wig onto my head. Never mind mentally to overcome the lassitude, the fatigue, the weariness about my situation and the many more cycles to come just to get myself doing what I felt I still needed to do each day. Now I was not only battling the thought that the cancer might not succumb to the treatment, but also becoming more aware that *I* might succumb to the treatment.

I had been having Adriamycin and Cytoxan since the week before Christmas, and we were now past Presidents' Day. Being halfway through was a milestone, but from the glass-half-empty perspective, I still had another twelve weeks to go, six cycles of another chemotherapy drug, Taxol. Dr. Liu and Claudine both tried to comfort me by telling me that the Taxol was less toxic and that I would, as oncologists like to say, "tolerate it better." My hair would start to grow back once I was off the Adriamycin and Cytoxan, and I would start to feel more energetic. They were full of oncologist cheer and optimism, traits they had to perfect, I was sure, as they encouraged thousands of women to cross the finish line. I focused on their positive projections and anticipated an easier road for the next twelve weeks.

That was before Marc Lippman got involved. And maybe saved my life.

As John gave talks or met with people about the treatment of gastrointestinal cancer, he would allude to my breast cancer and say that he had to schedule his time away from Washington around my treatments. This would lead, of course, to people expressing sympathy and asking questions. Many of these people naturally knew a lot about cancer, so their responses were more specific than those of the layperson. This could be a discomfiting side effect of my intimate relationship with a world-traveling, lecture-giving oncologist during treatment; it seemed as if the entire cancer world knew of my diagnosis.

I knew how bad my situation was. I had taken to Googling "triple-negative breast cancer" every week or so. Website after website said the same thing: very aggressive, poor outcomes, hard to treat, high rate of recurrence. I felt sick. I should never do that again, I thought. And yet for the next few years, like a moth drawn to fire, I would Google it again and again. Did it really say that? Had the descriptions on the Internet (and hopefully in reality as well) gotten any better? But they continued to give the same dire prognosis, and I repeatedly searched, felt sick, and swore not to do this again, despite the inevitable torment.

It was a bit odd, I suppose, when I actually lived with "Dr. Google," as physicians like to refer to this phenomenon of searching for medical information on the Internet. John wasn't experienced in breast cancer and particularly not in this relatively recently discovered form. I also knew he wasn't going to say the devastating things the Internet said— not the unreliable sites, of course, but even the reliable sites had very little good news to offer patients like me. He didn't want to discourage me or himself. We had plans for the time after the children were gone, after retirement, and my death really would mess them up.

My situation did work its way through the oncology pipeline, though, which turned out to be a plus. One day John called me to tell me he had just received an e-mail out of the blue from his former boss at the Lombardi Cancer Center, breast cancer specialist Marc Lippman, who recommended that I try platinum therapy.

John was familiar with platinum-based drugs and told me that he too thought they might be a good idea at this point. The aggressiveness of triple-negative breast cancer terrified us, and the studies on the use of platinum-based drugs in metastatic triple-negative breast cancer looked as if they were successful so far. No one had published a study on platinum-based drugs in localized triple-negative breast cancer like mine, but at least to me, the drugs seemed as if they were worth a try.

John mentioned our conversations to Dr. Liu, which must have put her in a difficult situation. First, John was her boss. No matter how hard we all tried to act as if there was nothing other than the doctor-patient relationship between us, how could she and John ignore the work relationship they had? John tried hard in appointments to act like just a caregiver and husband. I'm sure that she tried to ignore the elephant, who happened to be in charge of her reviews, sitting in the room. Second, Marc Lippman had been the director at Lombardi and was one of the most prominent and smartest breast cancer doctors in the United States and perhaps in the world. Dr. Liu potentially faced going against *his* recommendation. Dr. Liu is, however, the consummate professional, and if she was uncomfortable with the recommendation, she never let on.

My adding a platinum-based drug was going to have the additional disadvantage for John and Dr. Liu of my exiting the clinical trial. The point of clinical trials is for scientists to learn what treatments are effective and what aren't, and to move treatment of cancer forward. But getting patients to join clinical trials is difficult, and I'm sure that having me pull out was not the conclusion Dr. Liu was hoping for. By switching to the platinum-based drug, I was going to remove my data points from the results.

Despite all this, after going over the potential risks and benefits of changing course, she told us that we should do what we wanted. I still wasn't sure what the right answer was, so I took advantage of having yet another breast cancer expert in my orbit and called Claudine. Claudine danced around the issue a bit. She also didn't want to tell me what to do, a seeming code of conduct among oncologists, and she was, I think, also uncomfortable about recommending that we go in a different direction from that set out by Dr. Liu, Claudine's colleague and, in a sense, protégé. She acknowledged recently that she really struggled with what the change in treatment would mean for Dr. Liu, to have her plan contradicted by Marc Lippman, and that contradiction in a sense supported by Claudine. At the time, however, she confirmed that there was evidence of platinum drugs showing effectiveness in combating metastatic triple-negative breast cancer, which argued in favor of my trying it.

I wanted to do whatever I could to cure myself. Marc Lippman knew a lot, so I was inclined to do whatever he recommended. There were additional potential side effects with another drug in the mix, but I hoped I was going to be increasing my chances of a full cure as well. And yet I felt bad. Over the years, John had drummed into me how important clinical trials were. This one sounded promising, and I was Mrs. Dr. John Marshall, the head of clinical research at Lombardi Cancer Center. It wasn't a good look for John, not that he ever said or implied anything to that effect, but I felt some responsibility to carry the flag for clinical research.

In the end, though, I had to do what I felt the most confidence in. The idea of throwing every drug possible at this cancer appealed to me. John seemed supportive of adding the platinum drug as well, so in early March, I told Dr. Liu that I would like to come off the SWOG study and add a platinum drug to my chemotherapy regimen. She recommended that I have a combination of Carboplatin (a platinum-based drug) and the previously planned and standard-of-care treatment, Paclitaxel (Taxol), which would be administered once a week for three weeks and then a fourth week off. I would have that regimen for four cycles, so four more months and twelve more infusions. In retrospect, I realize that Dr. Liu was also put in the position of having to research what platinum drug to use and how to administer it to me in a way that was effective but safe. There was no standard of care for platinum drugs being used as adjuvant therapy for triple-negative breast cancer. I was going to be a trial of one.

At this point, I had had six separate infusions of a drug that was damaging my veins, and getting an IV started was becoming more difficult for the nurses and more unpleasant for me. Now I faced twelve more IVs. I started to rethink my decision not to have a mediport implanted. I talked to John and Dr. Liu about it, and their attitudes could be summed up as "Why didn't you do it sooner?" I scheduled the procedure to be completed before my next infusion and before my upcoming CT scan, which also would require an IV.

John took me to the interventional radiology unit of Georgetown Hospital at 7:00 a.m. on March 8. It was an outpatient procedure, and I should be home by lunch. They "twilight" you so that you aren't completely out, but you are out enough not to know what really is going on. They made a small incision on the left side of my upper chest, just under my collar bone, which is where the port was implanted, and they made an even smaller incision on the left side of my neck so that they could insert the tube from the port into the subclavian vein.

On March 12, 2007, I had a CT scan, this time with no need to start an IV! I did have to start all procedures now by going to the infusion unit first to have the port "accessed," which meant about fifteen minutes of numbing cream taped to my chest over the port, then having the small needle inserted and a shot of saline to clear the port. It had to be done in the infusion unit each time because only the chemotherapy infusion nurses were trained to do this. This added time to everything I did at the hospital and required an appointment with the infusion unit so they would know I was coming.

I hated having scans. I could put most of what might or might not be happening in my body to the back of my mind for much of the time except when it was about to be photographed, and someone was going to look at that picture and tell me what they saw. I was too nervous to read in the radiology waiting room, so I had started doing the *Washington Post Sunday Magazine* crossword at times like these. It required enough mental work and focus that it calmed my nerves somehow, so I sat there, waiting to be called back, a small tube taped to my chest, eyes bowed to my crossword.

The routine was familiar now: A medical assistant cheerily escorted me to a small changing room and gave me a gown. I changed and waited there with my crossword in one hand and my pen in another until I was called into the scanner room. Almost always after the scan was completed, one of the radiologists would check the scan and be sure that it was readable and didn't require another look. They were kind enough to tell me immediately that things looked good on the first quick look, but that my oncologist would give me the full results. I was seeing Dr. Liu right after, so I knew I wouldn't have to wait long to get the news from her.

The appointment with Dr. Liu was part of the routine on my treatment days, for her to go over the bloodwork required before every infusion and tell me about what this next adventure in chemotherapy would look like. It was two weeks since my last infusion of Adriamycin and Cytoxan, but this was going to be a different, as Taxol can produce a serious allergic reaction in some people. She began with the good news that nothing appeared to have changed since my last CT scan the preceding November. The lung nodule didn't look any different, which was great news because it meant that it was unlikely to be cancerous, but rather an old and stable defect of my body.

New information in hand, I returned to the infusion unit to begin the new regimen. Because of the potential for a serious allergic reaction to Taxol, it has its own protocol for the first administration. John came upstairs with me rather than his usual sending me on my way. Perhaps he was more apprehensive about the possibility of my having an allergic reaction than I realized.

When John and I arrived at the infusion unit, the unit secretary greeted us with her usual big smile and escorted us to a room. I unpacked my bag of entertainment for the day and settled onto the bed. John wandered around the unit, checking on his patients and reading an e-mail or two or twenty. After about fifteen minutes, Mercedes came in to give me a dose of Benadryl to mitigate any allergic reaction to the Taxol. I took it in pill form because I am sensitive to the soporific effects of antihistamines. This was later proven to be a good choice since for one cycle, I accidentally received the IV version and went from sitting up and talking to sound asleep in about fifteen seconds; it took me hours to wake up properly!

John wandered back in. Claudine happened to be on the infusion unit checking on a patient of hers, and she stopped by to say hello. When she realized that I was getting my first infusion of Taxol, she also decided to stay to see how it went. My anxiety began to build as John and Claudine casually expressed an interest in hanging around. It began to appear that this threat of an allergic reaction was a bigger deal than I had thought, and I asked tentatively what could happen. "Well, you could get a rash or itching," Claudine said. "Or you could go into anaphylactic shock," John added helpfully. I'm sure that wasn't the precise exchange, but that was what I heard. I had taken enough kids with peanut allergies to the zoo and restaurants to know that anaphylactic shock was pretty close to death unless someone acted quickly with an injection from an EpiPen. I began to shiver in anticipation. I was grateful that Claudine and John were there to keep me company and distract me from what was coming, and I knew that Mercedes was very experienced. I reminded myself that I was in good hands. Surely no one had ever died during an infusion of Taxol at Georgetown.

Mercedes soon reappeared with the bag of Taxol and what turned out to be a fishing tackle box, which contained medications pre-measured and pre-loaded to combat an allergic reaction immediately if I had one. Ominous. But amusing too. You would think there would be specific medical equipment to contain this artillery, rather than a piece of sporting equipment.

Mercedes started the IV and stepped back across the room. She stood bracketed by Claudine and John in their white coats, lined up facing me, standing with their muscles tensed. They all stared at me worriedly while I looked apprehensively back at them, each of us on tenterhooks as we waited to see if something bad was going to happen as the Taxol dripped slowly into my subclavian vein. The fishing tackle box actually was appropriate; I felt like a fish in a tank as they studied my every movement. I kept running internal surveys of my body: Was I itchy? Did I feel woozy? Could I breathe properly? Oh no, I can't breathe! Wait, take a deep breath. I guess I *can* breathe. But what about now? Still breathing. I focused on deliberate in and out, trying not to send myself into an anxiety attack.

As the minutes ticked by, Claudine, John, and Mercedes gently joked about whether I looked conscious. I started to relax as each minute passed without any apparent ill effects. After about fifteen minutes, I looked unaltered, so everyone exhaled and resumed relaxed chatting, no longer their forced prattle. Mercedes slipped out with the dreaded fishing tackle box to get to her next patient. John and Claudine both bid me farewell and moved on to the rest of their days. I appeared to be surviving and not allergic to my first administration of Taxol, which was a relief. All those who had stood vigil were free to return to their normal activities, and I returned to mine, sitting on a hospital bed with deadly drugs being dripped into my subclavian vein while watching soap operas and game shows and doing crosswords.

CHAPTER 22

Chemo Does Its Worst

A s I started the Taxol/Carboplatin regimen on the second Monday in March, I thought I was doing pretty well. The parts of me that hurt were less painful thanks to the drop in the Adriamycin dosage over the last two cycles and the liberal use of NSAIDs. Unfortunately, I had developed a weird fluid-filled protrusion from my cornea in the lower corner of my right eye, which in yet another time-consuming visit to yet another specialist, my ophthalmologist diagnosed as possibly a conjunctival inclusion cyst, whatever the heck that was. He said it was best to leave it alone, and it should go away eventually. I could only hope it would. I was beginning to look more and more like a freak—no hair, no eyebrows, no eyelashes, a protruding cyst in my eye, pale skin, and a gait impeded by sore feet. All those physical aberrations were causing me to feel more dejected, depressed, and probably more irritable at home. Each new problem dragged me down mentally, both finding the problem and figuring how to make time to see yet another doctor.

All in all, though, I supposed I was bearing up pretty well, and at the end of March I had made it through a full cycle of the new drugs, three doses each week for three weeks and a week off. We had even gotten in a shortened spring break. I had my third Taxol and Carboplatin treatment on the last Monday in March, and then we packed the family in the car and spent a couple of quiet and peaceful nights in Shepherdstown, West Virginia. We visited Antietam and Harper's Ferry (because who *isn't* cheered up by Civil War sites?), and the kids played behind the hotel, in a setting out of *The Railway Children*, next to the Potomac River under a railroad bridge. I sat in the room and watched them out the window, smiling at their freedom from care and their camaraderie. We had some lovely dinners and enjoyed driving through the beautiful Maryland countryside. I rested, and John didn't have to prepare a meal for almost a week. We even visited with friends in Baltimore whom we hadn't seen in several years. It was an idyllic break for all of us, particularly in retrospect as I realize what plans my body was hatching to complicate matters over the next few weeks.

On April 9, I began the second cycle of Taxol and Carboplatin, but when I went in to have the second dose of this cycle a week later, my labs showed that my platelet count was seventy thousand per microliter of blood, the bottom of the normal range being one hundred fifty thousand. A low platelet count can lead to your blood failing to clot and thus easy bruising and unusual bleeding.[1] The lab results also showed that my absolute neutrophil (white blood cell) count was eighteen hundred per microliter, the bottom of the normal range for those being one thousand. If your neutrophil count is low, it indicates that your immune system is weakened and that you are at increased risk

---

1 "Thrombocytopenia (Low Platelet Count)," www.mayoclinic.org/diseases-conditions/thrombocytopenia/symptoms-causes/syc-20378293, September 29, 2019.

of getting a serious infection.[2] Because the Carboplatin is hard on the red blood cells and platelets, and because my platelet count was so low already, Dr. Liu decided to give me only the Taxol, not the Carboplatin, in the second dose. I weathered that round of chemotherapy and felt pretty good.

Once again, I didn't concede to the risks of infection but persisted in going out in the germ- and bacteria-infested world. I attended school events, softball and baseball games and practices, a horseback riding lesson, board meetings, the Suzuki violin festival—all full of risks to an immunocompromised person. I just wasn't interested in living a life confined to the house and dousing myself with hand sanitizer every five minutes.

Having blithely been in the world for the week and having had the previous week's dose of the Carboplatin held, I assumed it was smooth sailing ahead when on the morning of April 23, I showed up at George-town for my blood tests and my next dose of Carboplatin and Taxol. I had my port accessed and blood taken and then went to John's office, as I often did, to hang out someplace other than the infusion unit while I waited for my lab results to verify that I could have the next dose of chemo. I don't think it ever occurred to me that I might not be allowed to have my scheduled chemotherapy. Dr. Liu had gone over all the risks with me as she was required to do, and I had heard them, but like the mandatory briefings about the safety presentation on an airplane, it all seemed pro forma. I was well aware of the risks of chemotherapy from John's conversations with patients who had a fever, bleeding, or even incipient organ failure, and had to go to the emergency room to get

2 "Low White Blood Cell (Neutrophil) Counts and the Risk of Infection," www.cancer.org/content/cancer/en/treatment/treatments-and-side-effects/physical-side-effects/low-blood-counts/infections/infections-in-people-with-cancer/low-wbc-and-weak-immune-system.html, September 29, 2019.

admitted to the hospital because of the chemotherapy rather than the cancer. I appreciated that it was a delicate balance, but none of these dire scenarios would apply to me, I thought. Aside from the cancer, I had gone into this in excellent health, so I figured I could handle the damage that chemotherapy was doing to my body.

In some ways, I actually considered myself to be pretty lucky to have breast cancer rather than an internal cancer because the only surgery required was to scrape an essentially exterior part off my chest without affecting any of my functioning internal organs. I have seen my mother over the years as she has dealt with the aftereffects of having 60 percent of her colon removed, which has led to several hospitalizations that required a tube to be threaded through her nose, down her throat, and into her stomach to keep her stomach and bowels empty until her bowels "unwound." She even had to have surgery to remove adhesions, a buildup of scar tissue on internal organs, from the original colon cancer surgery. I was unlikely to have such complications from my surgery, and I might have been overly sanguine about possible internal problems from cancer treatment.

I was sitting in John's office where he had that first fateful discussion with Dr. Liu five months earlier, but this time she called my cellphone to tell me that my labs were too low to have the final dose of the second cycle at all. My platelet count was now down to sixty-three thousand per microliter against a normal low of one hundred fifty thousand, and my absolute neutrophil count was down to seven hundred per microliter against a normal low of one thousand. The numbers were not good, and certainly not good enough to attack my cells further. I was devastated. I cried and whimpered. "Are you sure?" This was starting to sound like the conversation in November. Dr. Liu clearly felt terrible...again. "I'm really sorry. I wish we hadn't given you so much of the Adriamycin and Cytoxan. We've really beaten up your bone marrow. But we can't give you any more chemotherapy today. Could you come in and see me on Thursday so we can talk about what to do next?"

I wasn't happy, but it wasn't her fault, and there was nothing I could do about it. John clearly felt bad as well. It seemed like such a setback. So much of dealing with cancer for me was *doing something*, and now I was not going to be doing anything but waiting. What if I got sicker and ended up in the hospital? What if I couldn't do treatment anymore? "This happens all the time," he said. "My patients frequently have bone marrow issues and can't have treatment, but it's just a small setback, and your body will recover quickly." I wasn't sure I believed him. I knew he was trying to make me feel better and probably trying to assuage his own fears, but I don't like being coddled with platitudes, so I lashed out. "How do you know? Have you given this treatment before?" He had the good sense not to argue back, just to take me home and leave me be. I sat in the family room, feeling defeated and scared and like a failure.

That Thursday, John and I returned to an examining room at Lombardi with me on the patient table, John on one side and Dr. Liu on the other, in charge. She expressed her regret again about the six cycles of the Adriamycin and Cytoxan required by the clinical study and what they had wreaked in my bone marrow. She gave me two options going forward, stating that the current dosage of Carboplatin and Taxol was no longer possible because of the harm the Carboplatin was doing. She said technically she could reduce the doses of both, but she thought that might not be enough chemotherapy to be effective. Instead, she recommended either dropping the platinum drug altogether and just taking Taxol for two more cycles or substituting cisplatin for Carboplatin because cisplatin is less associated with low platelet counts. As she explained her reasoning, I was not really comprehending the details, since this was fundamentally a decision based on science and physiology.

John sat listening intently, but he was not going to tell me what to do; the decision was mine. I opted for the change in platinum drug because I still believed that the more I threw at this, the better chance I had at survival. Besides, since Marc Lippman said I should have it, maybe it was the secret sauce that was going to save me. Dr. Liu thus decided to slightly lower the dosage of both the Taxol and the cisplatin and to change the cycle from once a week for three weeks with the fourth week off to once a week for two weeks and then the third week off for two more cycles. In addition, she would have me receive a Neupogen injection each Thursday, Friday, and Saturday before each Monday treatment to maintain my neutrophil counts and to try to avoid further delays in treatment. Hurray, more quality time with my husband giving me shots!

One of the disadvantages of cisplatin is that it can be quite damaging to the kidneys, so a significant amount of saline is required to be infused both before and after administration to clear as much cisplatin as possible out of the kidneys quickly. This lengthened my days at the hospital significantly. The new protocol would involve more than two hours of saline with a diuretic in it, fifteen minutes of an anti-emetic drug, twenty minutes of Pepcid to prevent a reaction to the Taxol, an hour and ten minutes of Taxol, a little over an hour of cisplatin, and then two more hours of saline, this time with magnesium sulfate to boost my magnesium levels, which could be diminished significantly by the cisplatin. That's a total of almost seven hours of just infusions. Cisplatin was one bad drug! Maybe the cancer cells would run screaming or die on the spot when confronted with it.

Now, instead of arriving at the hospital at 1:00 p.m. and staying until 5:00 or 6:00 p.m., I had to arrive at 9:00 a.m., which actually meant 7:30 or 8:00 a.m., since that was John's usual arrival time for work. It was only two out of three Mondays, and we were nearing the end, but chemotherapy was now a full-day affair. I hadn't given up much in my day-to-day life until now. I remained on all the boards and committees I served on, continued teaching Sunday school, drove Charlie and Emma wherever they needed to be (which was *a lot* of places), attended their performances, lessons, and games, walked the dog, made lunches, cooked dinners, did the grocery shopping, and handled the family finances. The only day I really conceded to cancer treatment was the day with the needle actually in me, and that was fine by me. People asked me frequently why I didn't give things up, assuring me that everyone would understand, but I didn't want to. Maintaining my normal life was crucial to my state of mind. I've never been good at sitting around. I can do it for a day here and there, and my chemo days provided that, but otherwise I wanted to keep at it, whatever "it" was. I gain much of my self-esteem and happiness from accomplishing things and being a part of what's going on, so I worried that if I gave things up, I would become depressed. What was I going to do without my usual activities? Sit around and think about dying? I thought that would be worse than soldiering on through days I didn't feel so good.

Unfortunately, the cyst in my eye had not gone away, and I was finding it more and more annoying, not to mention embarrassing with my spiky wig and no eyebrows. Look Good Feel Better had not taught me how to cover up the eye cyst. Then a quarter of my right eye filled with bright red blood. (This was *really* not lovely.) I panicked and called the ophthalmologist's office immediately. They are always swamped, but they fit me in that afternoon, and John met me in the doctor's office to see what they thought and whether they could do anything. I didn't want to go out in public at all now, and I didn't know how long this might last. Maybe forever.

After what seemed an interminable time in the waiting room, I with my eyes downcast so no one could see what a freak I was, a young medical technician called us back. She went over my history, looked at my eye from afar and said, somewhat uncertainly, that she didn't know what it was, but that one of the ophthalmology residents would be in to see me. All of a sudden, I felt something dripping down my face. I didn't know what had happened, but the look of horror on the technician's face didn't bode well. I looked at John, and he said triumphantly, "I think it just burst!" The cyst had ruptured while we were contemplating the next steps, and a small stream of red blood was dribbling down my right cheek. No wonder the tech looked horrified. She handed me a tissue to clean myself up, and when I saw the blood, I was disgusted too, but also relieved. At last, a problem seemed to be resolved. After the tech left, a resident and the doctor came in and assured me that the issue should be at an end. John announced that the technician was a genius and had solved my problem without even touching me. The cyst healed up, never to reappear, and I had scarred one medical technician for life. On the other hand, she had been deemed a genius, so maybe that was compensation.

CHAPTER 23

All We Are Left With

If I could have one day with my mother again, I would ask her to share every memory; tell me her deepest thoughts, loves, favorite foods, and favorite season; what bugged her the most about Dad, David, Elizabeth—yes, OK, even me. My father is a great storyteller, but he tells the same stories over and over, except those rare times when we bring up a topic that breaks loose a new narrative we've never heard before. He leans into the joyful tales, rarely touching on pain or sadness. His dislike of remembering the bad stuff might be genetic. I too have a selective memory for the good stuff, which has proved to be a useful approach in my career as an oncologist.

In the end, our memories are who we are, all that remain. They define us. Why do we keep some, shake off others, treasure a few, share some, never share the dark ones? Until she died, my mother was our historian, and when she died, so too did a large set of life events, details that if they had been shared, repeated, and drilled into the family lore, most certainly would have altered my life's path.

Just this past year, out of the blue, my mother's younger sister, Ann, sent me a stack of old letters and clippings she had saved from my childhood. She admitted being a bit of a hoarder, maybe just a pack rat, and was overcoming one of her neuroses by finally getting rid of stuff. She too was diagnosed recently with cancer, so maybe she was clearing out her house while she still could. Many of the items were of little interest, but I appreciated that she handed off the keep-or-pitch decisions to me. In the stack were old thank-you notes my siblings and I wrote long ago, likely at my mother's insistence if not at gunpoint. There were yellowed newspaper clippings about my mom, including a story about a fashion show fundraiser in memory of my mother for the Jane S. Marshall Scholarship, with no mention of a school or purpose. I wondered if any money was raised and if anyone received the intended support.

Next were a few letters my mother had written to my aunt, still in their envelopes, postmark preserved. I read through them, struggling with my mother's bad penmanship. In one, she is "chatting along" about us kids, her busy life, and then without breaking stride, without any sadness or requests for sympathy, she explains her need for two thousand more rads of cobalt radiation to the growing lymph nodes behind her stomach and along the aorta. The first three thousand rads did not do the trick, she confides. She briefly laments her unyielding follicular lymphoma and then resumes her updates on life in Lexington, as if what she just shared was no different than whether I went to camp that summer.

Cobalt radiation is no longer used as it is too imprecise and too toxic. Radiation to the abdomen causes extreme nausea and fatigue. It can cause stomach ulcers and diarrhea, and it can lower blood counts. Back then, there were no good anti-nausea meds and little supportive care. You simply had to be sick, badly sick, miserable, no appetite, weak. It was awful.

A few images of her being seriously ill remain permanently seared into my hard drive. She was scrawny with wispy hair. One day we found her curled up in a ball in the corner of our parents' bedroom, having bled from what I now assume was her vagina. I don't remember ever being there to help her, much less being asked. Sure, I was around. I remember going to radiation appointments after school. I am pretty sure I did not go any extra miles to clean up after myself, not to fight with David, to check on her, to simply sit next to her and hold her hand. I lived my life. That seemed to be what was expected of me. We were to keep pushing forward and not dwell on cancer. We would not consider death. I cannot recall any discussion of her possible death.

The next letter in Aunt Ann's stack was typed and carefully edited, including some small handwritten additions. My aunt had put a yellow sticky note on the outside of this particular one to disclaim the "squabble" my mother referred to, and by the way, this was written a few months before she died. The entire letter was a typical post-family argument reconciliation. It was clear that my mother had been stewing on whatever had happened between them, having lost two nights' sleep worrying over it.

Reading between the lines and knowing both personalities, I think that my aunt must have been bugging my mother about how "not clean" she kept our house and how "bad" she was as a hostess. I imagine Mom simply could not take it anymore. She must have blown up. There was mention of a phone call that my mother did not want to pick up, but when she did, she apparently was short with my aunt. Mom said she was tired. She had taken on so much, including serving on the committee to hire a new preacher at our church. She and Dad had just returned from driving around visiting preachers in North Carolina. She commented on liking the triangle area, including Durham, where I would one day go to college and meet Liza. She clearly needed to get a lot off her chest about their family relationships. But having done that, she moved on and said she was looking forward to some nice events a few months ahead.

Up to that point, I had been reading the letter aloud to Liza and Emma, an engaged audience, mostly chuckling at the normalcy of it all and the joy of the precious new insights I was getting into my mother's life and my past. But when I read the part that referred to the summer ahead, I choked up. I realized that she would be dead by then. In fact, she had very little future ahead. For all I know, this might be the last thing she ever wrote.

How could she not have known that she would be dead in three months? Why would she have used her energy for finding a new preacher for our church and not on us? How come she used her diminishing energy and time to write this letter to her sister, who drove her crazy, instead of writing one to me? Maybe she did, and it is in some box somewhere, lost in one of the moves over the years. Maybe she wanted to but could not bring herself to do it. Maybe talking about death and the end of her life would undermine her own need to push forward and sustain hope. Maybe her calling to God was stronger than to us, and she knew we would be OK in the end. I'll never know. Not unless I get that one day with her I so long to have.

To this day, I feel a void, an irretrievable part of me that was lost when my mother died. No good-byes, no final instructions to be good, don't hit your sister, study hard, go to church. No closure. Just poof, she was gone. While I still often "feel" my mom around me and sense her presence at unexpected times, I have not "heard" her. In church, I still listen for her voice, hoping for whispered instruction, some expression of pride. During Communion, the Protestant white bread and grape juice kind, without fail I speak to her and get no response. Maybe there is no God, maybe no heaven.

And yet I always seem to see and hear my former patients who have died. They are my omnipresent failures, talking to me, giving advice. I see their faces in people I see at the mall and the airport. But never my mother. I probably could use a bit more therapy—maybe a lot more. She must be watching over me because how else could I account for all my good fortunes in life? Still, I listen but hear nothing. My mother's sudden absence, even though everyone else knew it was coming, is still painful. If I can, I don't want any other kid to have to live life with this emptiness, these unanswered questions. I translate this void into an arguably crazy and emotionally dangerous behavior at work.

When I signed up to be an oncologist, I thought that most of my patients would be older, past parenting. But due to unclear forces, we are seeing an unexplained dramatic increase in younger people with GI cancers, particularly colon cancer. Now I have a fairly large population of patients in their twenties, thirties, and forties. Most are parents with children. I both love and dread taking care of these patients. They have many unique issues not shared by the older age group. For example, they have no choice but to keep working, for money, maybe for sanity and hope. They have to keep parenting and raising their families. While everyone wants to live longer, the younger patients really want every day they can get. They will do anything possible for even one more minute; each additional day is another chance to see kids grow, change, and mature. They set landmarks based solely on their kids: graduating from college, high school, or sadly, sometimes kindergarten.

Fueled by my own issues of loss, I jump into the emotional firepit with my patients and their kids. I routinely ask about the kids. What do they know about the diagnosis and prognosis? How are they? Anyone acting out? How is school? Parents with cancer have so many balls to juggle that they often "don't get around to" focusing on the impact on the children.

I have one couple who still, after one parent's having had metastatic cancer for many years, have yet to tell their teen children anything. That's right, nothing. No cancer here at all. I have been pounding on them to bring their kids up to speed, but the parents are afraid this will only make matters worse. I am more worried about those kids than I am about the parents. The kids are the ones who will be altered forever by this secret. Trust me, I know. Honestly, I hope that those kids have figured it all out on their own and are just playing along, but based on my own children's reaction, and mine many years ago, I fear they have not.

I have always shared my story about me and my mom and her cancer with my patients. I encourage parents to include the kids in the cancer process. I suggest they bring the kids to an appointment to meet me, see the place where the treatment is given, and ask questions of us. As patients get closer to the end of life, I often go one step further, walking the high wire above the emotional firepit. I offer to meet with the kids to discuss what is happening and what to expect. I do this to take the burden off the parents and to complement what children have already been told. Maybe I can lessen their imagination-enhanced fears. Sometimes the children of my patients are up to speed, but sometimes my meeting with them is the first time they have had a chance to talk to anyone about their parent's illness.

Yes, these meetings were my idea in the first place, but I really dread it when the parents accept my offer. Sitting across from serious, uncomfortable, sad-eyed children who deep down know what this is all about but are hoping beyond all hope that you are going to tell them something different costs me. Done right, the meeting can help ease pain, answer questions, and bring understanding. Done wrong, it can raise anxiety, disrupt family dynamics, and undermine relationships. The kids are there against their will, preferring to be almost anywhere else in time and place. Sometimes they hear a bit of what I am saying, but mostly they are focused on the overall shitty situation.

I tell them that their parents love them very much and have done everything they can do to get better in order to live one more day. I tell them that their parents are tired and need to rest. I tell them that I have been through what they are going through when I was their age, sharing, "I lost my mom to cancer when I was thirteen, so I know." With this they look up from their shoes or their phones right into my eyes, checking my sincerity and credentials. They see in my face that indeed, I do know. And often, this breaks the ice. One of them asks a question about the cancer, perhaps clarification about something they read online. Another asks about a treatment, and more questions come about pain. Why is Mom so tired all the time? Do I know when or how much longer she has? I do my best. I answer honestly but gently. I offer to answer anything else that comes up now or later. I give them the mournful oncologist look. I connect, and then I leave.

Walking away, shoulders slumped, head bowed, I exhale. Once out of sight, I shift my gaze up to heaven, and I ask God to look over this family, especially now. I ask God to look over me. Then I push forward, eyes focused ahead.

CHAPTER 24

The Merry Month of May

May 2007 was the culmination of many significant portions of our year and even of our lives: piano and violin recitals, playoff baseball and softball games, Youth Sunday at church, the end of the school year and its attendant duties (exams, teacher gifts) and festivities (end-of-the-year parties, team parties). Charlie would graduate from the school he had attended for nine years. For me, and really for all of us, it was the end of six months of chemotherapy and protracted days at the hospital. The good news was that since the cratering of my platelets and neutrophils, thanks to Dr. Liu's skillful handling of the chemotherapy treatments, I had tolerated the treatments well, with my levels rebounding and holding steady at healthy levels. That meant I was able to receive the last two cycles of Taxol and cisplatin as originally scheduled. My hair even started to come back in.

As I neared the end of chemotherapy, it was time to start working on the next step in my treatment, radiation, and to figure out where I would receive that. Georgetown had a very good radiation oncology group, but a well-respected and experienced radiation oncologist worked at a cancer center about seven blocks from where I had grown up in Alexandria, Virginia, and where my parents still lived. Radiation for breast cancer in those days was generally thirty-five treatments, given each weekday over six and a half weeks, so this was going to be a daily commitment. (I wonder if anyone has ever done a study on the effect on cancer patients' outcomes of radiation oncology offices taking the weekends off.)

The week of the beginning of my last cycle of Taxol and cisplatin, I met with Dr. Jane Grayson to discuss the plan for my radiation treatment, and all of a sudden I was just another patient. Radiation oncology is a much more precise science than medical oncology. In medical oncology, each treatment day is different. Your labs might be different, your side effects may have changed, all of which may lead to an alteration in what dosage of chemotherapy is actually given to you. Chemo patients can't proceed with their infusions until the administration has been approved by the doctor, which can happen only after he or she has reviewed the lab results to ensure that you are in good enough shape to receive the infusion. These drugs are toxic and dangerous, and they must be mixed very carefully and only immediately before they are used, so patients have to sit around and wait. If a lot of people are getting infusions that day, the process can be very slow, leading to long wait times, perhaps several hours between having labs taken and receiving the chemotherapy.

Radiation oncology offices, on the other hand, don't have to wait for blood to be taken and tested and results reviewed, nor do they have to wait for chemotherapy to be mixed, and anti-emetics and other medications to mitigate the effects of the chemotherapy to be infused. They take you back, give you a hospital gown, cycle you into the radiation room, administer the radiation, then send you home, and you do it all again the next day.

Dr. Grayson thoroughly examined the area where my right breast had been and explained that I was going to have thirty-five treatments, the last six of which would include a "boost" to the scar area, which I gathered was going to lower my chances of recurrence. Each treatment would take about fifteen minutes.

Then came the warnings. My skin would look like it had a bad sunburn, with redness, pain, and skin flaking off. She recommended a cream called calendula that was made from marigolds and was being used in France, but which the FDA had not yet approved specifically for radiation patients. It had been shown to reduce the effects of radiation therapy on the skin and was easy to get at health food stores and online. The downside was that it was in a petroleum jelly and required generous application to the upper-right quadrant of my torso and under my right arm several times a day, which was going to make a mess of my clothes. Dr. Grayson recommended that I purchase some inexpensive loose T-shirts to wear during the nearly seven weeks I would be undergoing radiation and for a while thereafter while the skin recovered.

Oversized T-shirts are not my usual style, so this was disconcerting. However, I had managed to get through six months of chemotherapy and about four months of baldness and lack of eyebrows and eyelashes, so I knew I could manage seven weeks of greased-up skin and sloppy T-shirts, too. I also would not be able to expose the radiated area to sunlight, as it was already going to be getting a *very* good tan that summer.

A likely major side effect of the radiation was fatigue, which would grow over time and would last for a few weeks afterward. Among the possible long-term effects were bone marrow suppression because the radiation enters the ribs as well as getting the surface of the skin, and later, cancers such as sarcomas. These risks were quite small, but piled on top of all the possible long-term effects of chemotherapy, you start to wonder how much longer you're going to live even if the breast cancer doesn't come back. Dr. Grayson told me that I was lucky to have the cancer in my right breast as that meant my heart would not be affected by the radiation. It's a complication for women who have cancer in their left breasts because radiation to the left breast unavoidably hits the heart. She told me that, oddly, cancer is 5 to 10 percent more likely to occur in the left breast than the right. Here was a percentage battle I had come down on the "right" side of for once, it seemed.

Radiation increases the risk of lymphedema, especially since I would receive radiation under my right arm, where the lymph nodes had been removed. She told me that she wanted me to see a lymphedema specialist there (even though I already had been through the whole protocol at Georgetown) to ensure that I knew all I needed to know. She also ordered me a lovely "gauntlet," a fingerless glove to wear with my compression sleeve on airplanes.

The coolest news was that I was going to get tattoos! Radiation oncologists tattoo the breast area with several small dots when they set up the radiation to delineate the exact area being radiated so that those administering the radiation each day know exactly how to direct the beams in order to get the full area that needs to be radiated without a millimeter more than is deemed necessary. A less cool side effect involved my future appearance. The radiation was going to make reconstruction rather more complicated. I hadn't yet had a discussion with anyone about the reconstruction of my removed breast. I had thought about it over the past few months, but not seriously since I was so enmeshed in treatment and knew it wasn't even an option for quite a while. Dr. Grayson recommended that I go ahead and speak to a plastic surgeon who specialized in breast reconstruction so that he or she would have some baseline before the radiation effects appeared.

There was a breast plastic surgeon at Georgetown, Scott Spear, who was known for taking complex cases, so I made an appointment with his office. He had a reputation of having little bedside manner and being a bit difficult, but he was well-respected for his skill, and if I was going to do this, I wanted the best outcome possible. There wasn't much point in going through surgery and recovery if I wasn't going to be happy with the way the breast looked afterward.

A week after I had met with Dr. Grayson—but before starting radiation—John and I met Dr. Spear, who I thought was actually quite sweet, with an incredibly kind and understanding office staff. Dr. Spear acknowledged ruefully that he tended to make people cry, so he was aware of his reputation. But he said it in such a tender and regretful way, he became more endearing. Someone who goes into non-cosmetic breast reconstruction must care about women who have been through breast cancer treatment and must want to make them feel better about themselves, not just make himself feel good about his accomplishments. I liked him and was happy to trust him with my treatment.

I had gotten used to sitting around in hospital gowns and having people look at my chest, but this was a bit more exposure than even I was used to. Dr. Spear asked me to take the gown off and eyed my chest critically. He then palpated the breast area and the underarm to see what the skin was like and how much there was to work with. He said the better option was to do what was known as a lat flap. With this surgery, a piece of skin and muscle is taken from your back on the side where the breast has been removed, and the blood supply is left attached to the piece of back and tunneled around the side and under the arm, where it then replaces the skin already there with the muscle providing the "heft" to the breast, so to speak. I was hesitant about this surgery because I am somewhat athletic—I enjoy golf and tennis in particular—and stubbornly right-handed. I didn't want to diminish my abilities to beat my husband at tennis with my wicked cross-court forehand or to outdrive him off the tee. Also, it was going to mean two places on my body that would be cut into and then sutured, meaning a greater risk of infection and more work to heal.

I apparently did not have enough belly fat for the use of abdominal tissue, a TRAM flap, to replace the breast tissue. This was the most popular form of reconstruction because you get a tummy tuck out of it, too! I wasn't enthused about that one either because it also required taking muscle, and I felt strongly about not losing muscle in my abdomen. My remaining option was an implant. Dr. Spear warned me that these are difficult to do on women who have had radiation because the skin isn't very healthy, and the chances of infection or poor healing are increased. They also can require two surgeries because a tissue expander is implanted first and slowly "inflated" with fluid over several months to stretch the skin out, and then the expander is replaced with the permanent gel- or silicone-filled implant. He said he would consider trying to do it with one surgery to limit the need for the radiated skin to heal repeatedly, but even then, the likelihood of it working was only 75 percent. He could sense my reluctance about cutting into any other part of my body and said he would evaluate the options after radiation was over in September.

Dr. Spear's practice was to have photos of women's breasts taken at every stage of the process for research purposes. He actually had a professional photographer on staff who took all of these pictures in a nice little photo studio in the office. It felt completely normal until it didn't, when I had to take the gown off and pose straight on to the camera plus once with each shoulder to the camera to get the full view. While I'm not especially modest, I'm not an exhibitionist either, so I felt uncomfortable. In my one-breasted state, I was more self-conscious about being seen naked than I had been. The photographer was the only person I came across in the entire process who treated me rather brusquely. She was efficient, though, and I was soon dismissed.

My visit to Dr. Spear came the day after my last chemotherapy treatment. There was no big celebration, but lots of smiles and congratulations plus some sadness. Having chemotherapy was a bit like pregnancy. You visit the doctor frequently; you get to know each other; you know all the staff, and they know you, so you start to feel as if you are all best friends. Then it's over, and I felt bereft. I loved Dr. Liu and Mercedes, along with all the people in the Lombardi clinic and the infusion unit. We'd had many lengthy conversations about our lives and our opinions on all sorts of topics, including sports teams, politics, and our favorite vacation spots. We had been through Christmas, New Year's, Martin Luther King Day, Valentine's Day, Presidents' Day, spring break, my birthday, other people's birthdays, Easter, Passover, Mother's Day, even Memorial Day, which was the day before my last treatment. You can't help but feel that you know people pretty well after that. It was hard to say good-bye. However, it wasn't to be forever as I had signed up for yet another clinical trial, which dulled the sadness and nostalgia. Lurking beneath it all was the knowledge that if my cancer returned, I would be back.

As for my physical state, my blood levels had rebounded, but I had started to become more fatigued. Also as expected, I began to develop some tingling in my fingers and toes, a side effect of both Taxol and platinum-based drugs. However, it wasn't severe, and I managed to keep going at a pretty normal pace.

As we approached the end of chemotherapy, Dr. Liu offered me another clinical trial, one that would require taking a bisphosphonate, a drug that many menopausal women were taking then to prevent the loss of bone density and to treat osteoporosis in the hopes of preventing "the old woman's curse," hip fractures, down the road. There had been some indication that these drugs seemed to have a protective effect on bones for patients whose primary cancer was of the bone. An IV form of bisphosphonate, Zometa, already was being used in patients who had prostate or breast cancer with bone metastases. Dr. Liu reminded me that there was no way to know whether the cancer cells from my right breast had made it through my bloodstream to other parts of my body despite all the chemotherapy, and the goal of this study was to try to make the bone an inhospitable environment for cancer cells. The study had three arms this time, two that required taking a bisphosphonate pill every day for three years and one that was given via IV every four weeks for the first six months, then once every three months after that for thirty months.

There was one possible side effect that concerned me, osteonecrosis of the jaw. For some people who are on the drug, instead of healing from dental surgery in a normal way, the bone in their jaw starts to die. The study required that I pass a dental exam before I could take part in the trial. Osteonecrosis of the jaw sounded horrible, and considering the mouth problems I already had, I was terrified about adding a drug that might feed on that vulnerability. But, as many cancer patients will tell you, the idea of stopping all treatment for your cancer is even more terrifying. I didn't want to stop infusing anti-cancer drugs because it felt like surrendering, allowing the cancer to find a foothold and to grow. Thus I signed up for the trial and three more years of "doing something" rather than "doing nothing."

I was "randomized" to the arm of the trial that used the IV, and I had my mediport, so I was outfitted for that. I had to visit the infusion unit once a month anyway to have the port flushed out, so it wasn't going to change my life much. I very much wanted to keep the port until I was sure that I was out of the woods cancer-wise because if I did have a recurrence, I didn't want to get the port reimplanted.

The port became a kind of talisman. As long as I had it, I was prepared for the worst, like taking an umbrella with you to keep it from raining. I had some other talismans and good luck charms that seemed to have stood me in good stead through chemotherapy as well. I had made it through without an admission to the hospital or even an emergency room visit—no fevers or infections despite my depleted immune system and my insistence on maintaining my normal life. My good fortune was clearly because of the beads one of John's fellows had given him for me, which I wore every day during treatment; a picture of an unidentified saint another fellow had given John for me, which I hung on the mirror over my dresser and remains there to this day; and the black cat that crossed my path every morning while I was walking the dog, then disappeared as soon as I was done with treatment.

May 2007 ended with Charlie's graduation from Alexandria Country Day School. My in-laws came into town for the big event, and we had plans for a celebratory dinner. A few days before graduation, the head of school told me that the president of the Board of Trustees was going to have to be away for graduation. The president traditionally handed out diplomas to the graduating eighth-graders, but they thought it would be nice if I filled in as a member of the Board of Trustees since my son was in the graduating class. I was flattered and quickly accepted. I then proposed a dramatic move to my family. Would it be OK if I didn't wear the wig? I was mostly bald with smooth, soft baby-like hair coating my head, but everyone in Charlie's class and on the school faculty knew I had no hair under that wig, and it no longer felt like me. At the same time, I realized that not wearing the wig would be a public announcement of all we had been through over the last school year, and this event wasn't about me. I wasn't looking for attention or sympathy, nor did I want to embarrass Charlie on a day that was about celebrating him. He, however, kindly and graciously said he was fine with my going "top down."

As I stood on the stage, shaking the hands of all these young people I had known for so many years, I felt beautiful and almost me again. Was I really over the worst? Was I cured?

CHAPTER 25

Radiation

No one mentioned how hard getting set up for radiation would be, but it was the worst experience of my entire cancer treatment. On June 4, 2007, I arrived at the radiation oncology suite, and after I changed, a medical technician led me to the radiation room, where I got on the bare-metal treatment table, surrounded by the massive arms of a large radiation machine. The arms protrude from the core of the machine behind your head, and they pivot down and in so that they are eventually at a ninety-degree angle from the core, with the ends directly facing your body. The machine's four arms then rotate around the table to line up as needed. The goal is to make sure that the radiation hits only the intended target without radiating any other parts of your body. This requires repeated simulation of where the radiation beams will hit your body, and X-rays are taken periodically to show the radiation therapist what he or she actually is doing. After that, the radiation oncologist reviews the data. If it isn't completely correct, the machines are realigned to change how the beams hit the area to be radiated, and they go through the simulation, X-rays, and review again.

What all those adjustments mean for the patient is that you have to lie *completely* still for about an hour on a hard metal table in an awkward and uncomfortable position with nothing soft or padded in sight. (Those lovely warm blankets were only a distant memory here.) My radiation oncologist's treatment room had several panels on the ceiling with bucolic scenes of clouds and flowers as an attempt to distract from the enormous discomfort—nice effort, but pointless for me. The therapists and technicians tried to be soothing and sympathetic, but staying in one position for an hour was brutal.

I don't know how others may have found it, but my first radiation appointment made me cry, and it's hard to cry and remain utterly still. I lay there on my back, uncovered from the waist up, with my right arm over my head for more than sixty long minutes. My legs cramped, my skin crawled, and my toes itched. I thought I was going to scream or shake my leg or just get up and walk away. I managed to confine my deep distress and discomfort to tears running down my cheeks. Dr. Grayson came in toward the end and saw me crying, and she apologized for how long it was taking. It was so they could do the best job possible, she explained, which of course I knew.

I was never more relieved to be told that someone was done with a procedure on my body. There were still the tattoos to be applied, but we had marker spots where those were to go, so at least I could move a bit first. I took full advantage of that permission, bringing my arm back down alongside my body, stretching my legs, rolling from one side to the other, rubbing my neck, scratching my nose, and wiping the tears off my cheeks.

A young woman in scrubs came in with a needle and a small amount of blue ink. She dipped the needle in the ink and inserted it just under my skin at the top left corner of where my right breast used to be, the bottom left corner of the same area, and two under my right arm close to the back. These four spots would show the therapists where to line up the radiation beams each day so that the exact same area received radiation each time. I sport these tattoos to this day, and the one on the upper part of my breast does show when I wear lower-cut clothes. It's just a random blue dot on my chest, but a permanent memento of that difficult day.

After the traumatic set-up experience, my radiation treatment was a breeze—quick and precise. Still, worry crept in. I have resisted unnecessary X-rays for years, having read in all sorts of publications of the damage that every bit of radiation does to you. Here I was, high doses of radiation bombarding my skin and my insides for the next six weeks, never mind all the CT scans, mammograms, and MRIs I had received over the past year. What was going to happen to my skin even with Dr. Grayson's magic lotion? As radiation treatment started, my desire to dress nicely seemed to diminish, and all I cared about was keeping a constant coating of calendula lotion on. I knew that my only chance at having an implant rather than taking skin and muscle from elsewhere depended on keeping the skin that remained from my right breast in good enough shape to come through more surgery and to heal properly afterward.

After about two weeks of radiation, I noticed a funny red bump in the middle of the scar across my right breast area. Was this a local recurrence of the cancer or something less? Was I becoming a hypochondriac? Maybe I was one already. I showed it to John, who didn't know what it could be, although he said he didn't think it was cancer since my breast was receiving bolts of radiation each day. Dr. Grayson looked at it and recommended that I get Dr. Willey to have a look at it, too. I hurriedly and anxiously called Dr. Willey's office as soon as I got home, and then rushed to Georgetown.

Dr. Willey's nurse practitioner examined the bump and surrounding area closely. She wasn't quite as proficient as Dr. Willey at maintaining an aura of good cheer, but she did say that it was probably what is known as a "suture granuloma," which had developed around one of the original internal stitches and had been irritated by the radiation. Then she sent me down the hall for an ultrasound. Back to my favorite room, where I had had the biopsy that had led to the diagnosis of breast cancer. The radiologist took a quick look with his ultrasound machine and agreed that it looked like a suture granuloma to him, so back I went to the nurse practitioner for her to prescribe some antibiotics just in case there was any infection in the area.

In the end, it did turn out to be a suture granuloma, which Dr. Willey offered to remove. The problem was that I would have to stop radiation while the area healed, and she and I had concerns about doing that. We had our annual family vacation starting two weeks after I was due to finish radiation, and I knew I was going to be pushing it with the sun exposure so soon after being radiated. The thought of this annual tradition had kept me going through radiation, and I couldn't bear the idea of missing any of it myself or causing anyone else to miss it either. I was NOT going to mess this up.

Cancer follow-up waits for no man or woman or radiation treatment, meaning that several pieces of treatment and follow-up happen on top of each other. On the rushing train of cancer care, I had a routine follow-up CT scan on July 16, and I started the new bone drug trial on July 23. The CT scan didn't show any changes, for which I was extremely grateful.

I returned to the infusion unit at Georgetown on July 23, ready for my first Zometa infusion. Because they were short, I now had my treatment in one of the infusion rooms that had several infusion chairs. I was happy to be in a more social setting. The close proximity in the rooms allowed those of us in the infusion chairs to learn each other's stories, both cancer related and otherwise. The patients were a mixed group, from those holding powerful jobs and multiple cell phones to people arriving after multiple buses and trying to figure out how to keep the home fires burning. Some patients had caregivers with them while others were alone. Sometimes you could tell that people were alone both on the infusion unit and at home.

Mercedes came in to access my mediport, gave me a dose of Tylenol (I should have paid more attention here), hooked me up to a bag of Zometa, and fifteen minutes later, I was done. My infusion went smoothly, and I went merrily on my way.

The next day I woke up feeling like I had the flu. I shivered, I felt sick, I had a headache, and my bones hurt. I could barely get out of bed, but I had radiation, and there wasn't a choice. Fortunately Charlie and Emma were both away at camp, so I didn't have them to worry about. However, I couldn't drive, so I had to call my parents and ask if someone could pick me up, drive me to my radiation appointment, wait for me, and take me back home. My mother kindly acquiesced.

I slowly dressed myself and dragged myself into her car, feeling and acting like a limp rag. She seemed disturbed by my condition. I sat in the waiting room pathetically until I was called back to change. For some reason, there was a long wait that day before my turn on the radiation table. I sat in the changing room, shivering uncontrollably, trying to tuck myself into a ball on an uncomfortable metal chair. The tech asked me what was wrong and if I was OK, and I told her I was fine but that I had just had the first infusion of Zometa, and it was not sitting well. She immediately brought me a blanket to cover up while I waited. I had to muster great self-control not to shiver during radiation, but somehow I succeeded. I actually knew that this might happen; I had been warned that all of the things I was experiencing were possible side effects. The purpose of the Tylenol with the Zometa was to mitigate some of the symptoms, but it did not succeed.

Dr. Liu called later in the day to check in. She said that although this kind of reaction wasn't uncommon with the first dose, it was unlikely that the second dose would cause me to feel so sick. She recommended that I help myself by taking ibuprofen the day before, the day of, and the day after the next round and each succeeding round, plus a dose of acetaminophen at the time of the infusion. I took some ibuprofen, and it worked like a charm! I didn't have a problem again. At least not this problem.

I completed radiation treatment about a week later with a cheery sendoff from Dr. Grayson and her team. I was done with my treatment! It did feel momentous and scary. What was going to happen now? I realized that I felt at sea. Here I was, eight months after a diagnosis that had changed my entire life as well as my family's, eight months filled with multiple forms of assault on my body, countless doctor visits, and numerous tests. Now I was on my own, and I didn't know what to do with myself. I was proud and relieved to have made it to the end of treatment for a particularly aggressive breast cancer, but I felt bereft and alone, too. I had become accustomed to constant medical monitoring, and even though I wasn't out of the woods, I wasn't *doing* anything about it either. I didn't want to burden John with my problems any longer. I had used up my credit there for a lifetime, I felt. I was going to have to figure out how to become a survivor, and I was going to have to do it by myself.

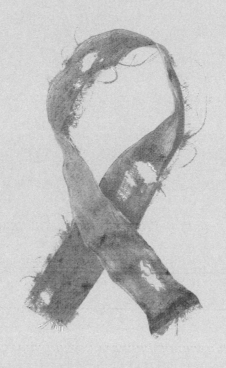

PART 6

If You Think Doctors as Patients Are Bad...

Lecture to Medical Students
Georgetown University Hospital
Washington, D.C.
January 2016

O K, you did a great job presenting that case, but I wanted to discuss something outside the normal curriculum. That patient you just presented to me was a retired doctor, right? How did that go? As a med student, did you find working up an experienced physician intimidating?

It is a well-established fact that doctors are the worst patients. We have our own ideas about things, and we have expectations of being treated faster and better than the regular, non-initiated "outsiders." OK, like royalty. Doctors change doses of their medicines, forget to take medicines, and think we don't need to follow orders. Orders are meant for regular humans, and doctors are not regular humans.

Guilty as charged. I regularly pull the "I am a doctor" line to receive special treatment. Sometimes when I am feeling less (or is it more?) obnoxious, I drop a few lines of high-tech doctor language, the surefire giveaway that I am in the business. It's my not-so-subtle way to notify the team that royalty is in the house!

But there's a flip side to this. Even today, thirty-plus years into practice, I still am a bit intimidated when asked to take care of other doctors. They know the language and the secret codes. Did I miss or fail to mention something that they know about? Are they testing me to see how much I know, or are they actually there to learn from me or have me help them? As I'm sure you are aware, I train doctors and am required to judge your performance. When I go to the doctor for myself, I cannot help but judge the "white coat" in front of me. Sometimes, when my own medical issue is not too serious, I go in undercover and pretend to be ordinary. I particularly like to do this when a resident or fellow or, better still, a medical student like you is involved in the visit, which in a teaching hospital like ours is the routine. It's a perfect chance to remind me what it is like from our patients' point of view—an opportunity to play "undercover boss."

I get almost all my medical care here at Georgetown. It starts with the incredible convenience but quickly extends to my love of the docs I work with, the friendliness of the staff, and my parking space. (This may be the most valuable asset in Washington.) I do not care much about my privacy. For me, all the positives of being treated by people you know far outweigh risking the loss of any remnant of privacy I have. Most residents don't know me, certainly not in a hospital gown, with skinny legs and dark socks hanging off the side of the exam table. To them, I am just some middle-aged Washington hypochondriac wasting their time.

You know the routine. You all go in as a scout to take the medical history and perform the physical exam. In just a few exchanges, I usually can figure out how far along you are in your training, even beyond the length of your white coat. Newbies like you are still mastering the basics. More senior residents exude the professionalism and knowledge one expects from a graduate. Don't worry; you will get there. Having gathered my information, they step out to talk in private with the attending resident, presenting my case and offering their summary of medical recommendations. Most residents are terrific—warm, bright, engaging, eager, everything you want in your doctor. They know what they know and, more important, what they don't know. But as in life, some are real jerks, not yet having learned how to talk to people, how to convey information, how to put people at ease. I am sure each of you could name a resident or two who fits this description. They somehow have developed an unearned air of superiority. To be honest, some residents, the *future scalpel throwers, never learn and are destined to grow up to be jerk attendings. I am secretly pleased to be incognito with them. After arrogantly taking my history, discounting my answers, performing a cursory physical exam, and generally pissing me off, the resident presents my case to the attending, who then discloses that I am the chief of hematology/ oncology. Oops, gotcha!*

If the attending physician is anything like me, he or she will have a touch of insecurity and uncertainty, wary of feeling judged by another physician. They hide the feelings, entering the exam room with an air of friendship and comfortable familiarity. We make small talk about work, the construction outside, and the new paint in the doctors' lounge, and then we get down to the business at hand. I don't want my doctors to be anxious, to feel judged. I want their best advice, their "A" game. Yes, secretly I hope that the arrogant resident is squirming, but only to teach a lesson. I want both of them to give me everything they've got.

Do I treat doctors differently? Absolutely. I try to provide them with a concierge level of service so often provided to me. But despite all my angst, in many ways, it is easier to treat doctors. You can use medical jargon. Doctors understand tests and the limitations of results. They have a sophisticated level of knowledge of their diagnosis and the treatment. They understand whatever we are telling them the first time, so there's no need to go over it again. (A real time-saver!) And having doctors pick you to lead their care team is a true compliment. Yes, they too may be seeing you for convenience and the free parking. But more likely than not, they have the choice of anyone in your field, and they have picked you.

Back to our patient: In the process of evaluating him, did anyone also interview his wife sitting at his bedside? You know sometimes caregivers are more important to talk to than the patient. Was she also a doctor? Have you run across a patient with a doctor as the primary caregiver yet?

Some doctor caregivers I have run into are quite memorable—for all the wrong reasons. I had a patient with an OB/GYN daughter who "attended" all of the patient's visits with me by phone. As I spoke, she was audibly clicking away on the Internet to check that everything I said was correct, jumping in as she uncovered something I had yet to mention. With a touch of insolence, she would ask why this was what I planned to do, then suggest that I must have forgotten this key point or that treatment. Maybe, for all my vaunted reputation, I was stumped. She said that she would check around with her colleagues, interrogating them about everything I did and said. After the visit, she would want to talk in the evening, to debrief, to see if I had learned anything new in the past five hours that might help her mom. I will never forget this woman. She's a constant reminder that arrogance and aggression in the quest for treatment are never a good idea.

Naturally, as caregivers, we all become protective; it's a key part of the job. Tasked with the new role of providing support, protection, and defense for our loved one, doctor caregivers work the system to their advantage. When scheduling an appointment for a critical test, only to find out that the next available appointment is three months from now, we "all-powerfully" pick up the phone, call the back line, and get an appointment for tomorrow. Hell, without a second thought, we will just walk into a colleague's private office, interrupting whatever he or she is doing, and ask for immediate help: "Sorry to disturb you, but my wife's problem is more important than anything you could possibly be doing right now."

While doctors have the best access, this phenomenon is not limited to doctor caregivers. Many of my non-doctor but well-connected caregivers pull just as many strings, call as many hospital presidents, and notify as many senators as they can to make sure we all know who is "in the house." Washington, D.C., can be a great place to practice medicine.

I never had to do any of this for Liza. I cannot recall ever flexing my privilege or cashing in a favor. The entire team did it all for us. People called us with times for scans, for labs, for pre-op testing. It all just rolled out in front of us with essentially no effort by either of us beyond showing up. Freed from this burden, we could focus on dealing with our kids, fulfilling our duties, telling others, and managing our own fears. There was no time spent on hold with radiology, no begging for an earlier time slot in the infusion unit, and no need to remind Liza's care team for a prescription refill. It felt automatic.

If I ever intimidated Dr. Liu (I was also her boss) or any of Liza's doctors, they never let on. I doubt whether anyone before and maybe since has ever received such amazing care. I know that all the other patients, the thousands that come through our doors every month, do not receive this level of service. I was both proud of our team and embarrassed by our riches. Our team had taken a large part of the caregiver role off my hands. They were not only making our burden lighter for Liza, but also making it lighter for me.

So why am I telling you all this autobiographical stuff? What does this have to do with your coming to this roundtable—aside from the free food, and I know that is not nothing. I am telling you this because during the time that my wife was sick, she received the kind of care that I believed every single one of our patients is entitled to. I made a deal with God and myself: If Liza got through her illness, I would provide the level of care she enjoyed for all our patients. It sounds like an excellent idea, right?

So now, let me ask you: Is my idea possible or a dream?

CHAPTER 26

Recovery

When did I feel recovered? These things are gradual; you don't wake up one day and realize that your life is 100 percent back to normal, or you feel as good as you are ever going to feel again. You just re-enter the fast lane on the jam-packed highway, and you don't have time to think about it on a daily basis. Every once in a while, however, the oncology machine tugs you back.

By the time we left for our family vacation in mid-August, I was getting some of my hair back, although I was obviously just post-cancer treatment or post-some-midlife crisis that had caused me to shave my head. We always *think* we know why a woman is bald, but we never can be *completely* sure. In summer clothes, I could see the scar under my left collar bone and the protrusion where the mediport sat. I could see the small scar on the left side of my throat where the mediport tube had been attached to the vein. I could even see (and feel, if I got up the nerve to touch it) the tube running under my skin from the vein in my neck down toward my collarbone. In a bathing suit or V-neck shirt, the top tattoo on my right breast area peeked out, as if I had stabbed myself with a ballpoint in a bizarre writing accident.

The most noticeable thing to me was how my chest looked in a bathing suit. I spent the spring trying to find a bathing suit that would take a prosthesis, but to no avail. My only option to cover up my imperfection (or at least the most obvious one) was to return to Nordstrom and have prosthesis pockets sewn into my bathing suits, as they had offered when I purchased my bras there.

When I wore the bathing suit, my flat chest seemed to shout its presence. On the left side of the neckline, there was a gentle curve and roundness from the front of my chest into the top of the bathing suit. On the right side, I was obviously flat from the chest wall all the way down. It almost looked concave. If I leaned forward, it was clear that I had no breast on the right, and if someone was indiscreet enough to stare at my chest from the left, it was noticeable that something wasn't quite right.

And yet I was relatively content with my body. I looked a bit strange in nightclothes (never mind naked), and I didn't love the way I looked in a bathing suit or low-cut clothes, but I had no desire to go back under the knife. I had been under medical care constantly since November of the preceding year, and my body was still not recovered, or at least not as recovered as I hoped to be from the assaults of the past eight months. I wanted to go through normal days and weeks and months and catch up with my life and projects.

Going to the beach could not have been a more perfect way to celebrate the end of my treatment. My mother's family had lived in the area for almost a hundred years, and I had spent every summer and Christmas there throughout my childhood. For all of us, it was a place where the cares of our world did not intrude, and if they did, we always found an answer to our problems as we dozed under an umbrella, caressed by the warm ocean breeze. This year was no different. We played golf and tennis, swam, walked on the beach, prepared family meals, laughed uproariously during rounds of charades and Password, visited with the local cousins and old high school friends of my mother's, and reminisced about summers past. It came to an end all too quickly, as it always did, but we were recharged and ready for the academic year to come, which would bring another big change: Charlie was going to boarding school.

Having your firstborn start high school is a big event, but having him leave the house as well felt seismic. We weren't new to the boarding school experience as John and I had both attended them. Charlie's new school, Episcopal High School in Alexandria, Virginia, was just a couple of miles away from our house and a few blocks from my parents' house. It was also the high school that John had attended. Charlie moved in and started school at the end of August, and our house was much quieter. Emma started middle school, and I returned at relatively full power to my domestic and volunteer jobs while figuring out how to attend every one of our children's sporting events.

On the one-year anniversary of my diagnosis, November 2007, since the treatment was done, we decided to have a party to thank the many people who had stepped in to support us over the last difficult year. We invited everyone who had helped us. It was life-affirming and happy. Yes, we knew that I wasn't out of the woods yet, but we knew how lucky we had been along the way to have had so much help and love and to have come through the year relatively intact. No matter what happened to me healthwise going forward, we needed to thank all of these people for everything they had done for us, and we needed to remember that each day really is a gift, no matter how trite that sounds.

It was now time to figure out how to heal my body *and* prevent my cancer from recurring. For anyone who has been diagnosed with a Stage 3 or above cancer, the threat of recurrence is terrifying and omnipresent. Will it appear in some other part of the body? Many breast cancer patients believed they were cured, and many years later they developed pain in their back or their neck. Thinking nothing of it, they had a CT scan "to be sure," and the scan showed recurrent breast cancer in the bone. Earlier in 2007, as I was switching from Adriamycin and Cytoxan to Taxol and Carboplatin, the news broke that Elizabeth Edwards, the wife of U.S. Senator John Edwards of North Carolina, who was running for president at the time, had broken a rib, and the scan had revealed "something suspicious" on another rib.[1] It turned out to be a recurrence of the breast cancer she had first been diagnosed with in 2004.[2] Her breast cancer was now incurable, and discussions turned to her ever-diminishing chances of making it five years.[3]

So I was well aware of the danger I was still in. I was doing my best to prevent bone metastases by going on the Zometa trial. Some people, I know, become vegetarian or give up alcohol or both, attend mind/body retreats, and join yoga classes. All of these efforts are admirable and effective in their own ways, but I'm a data person married to a cancer scientist, and no significant or repeated studies supported any of these activities as ways to prevent a recurrence of breast cancer. However, Dr. Liu had told me that there *was* strong scientific evidence that exercising regularly and not gaining weight were strongly linked to

1 "Edwards Says Wife's Cancer Has Returned," *New York Times*, March 23, 2007.

2 "Elizabeth Edwards Enters Second Cancer Fight," abc.news.go.com, March 22, 2007.

3 "Edwards Says Wife's Cancer Has Returned," op. cit.

lower recurrence rates for women with breast cancer, and she recommended that I try to get thirty minutes of moderate exercise five days a week.

It's harder than it sounds. Yes, I wanted to do everything to prevent my breast cancer from coming back, but every day there are new demands on your time and attention, and exercise has always made me feel a bit guilty. I am not good at doing things for myself, and I had just spent almost an entire year in which it had felt as if *everything* was about me. I wanted to repay some of that. I had maintained *some* exercise regimen while I was undergoing treatment, going to the gym in my cute little exercise cap to cover up my baldness, which I did for one session and then jettisoned it. We also had a dog, and I was the official family dog walker, so that got me out a couple of times a day. I knew that exercise would help my mental and physical well-being, but it was hard to sustain during treatment. Getting treated for cancer is incredibly time-consuming, and there were periods I physically couldn't work out because of the effects of chemotherapy.

After it was over, I resolved to resume regular exercise. I signed up for my free training session at the gym, which I knew was a sales gimmick, but I wanted to work with a trainer to get my strength back. I wanted someone who would be understanding about my risk of lymphedema and help get my right arm back to full strength or as close as possible, going beyond the limit of "lift nothing over five pounds." It seemed to me that, just in the way they tell you to keep things moving to move fluid out of parts of your body that are swollen or have suffered trauma, movement of my arm would keep lymphedema at bay, and not using it or pushing it might impede that endeavor.

To my good fortune, I was paired with a trainer who is still in our lives today. Said Bari began, as all trainers do, asking me about my physical condition, my goals, and my past attempts at exercise. But he went beyond that. He asked me about my surgery and lymphedema, and then he went home and researched it all so he could get me to my goals safely. I was able to return to exercise and am stronger and fitter now than I was before treatment. We blew by the five-pound limit on my right arm and loosened the scar tissue under my arm, but only because he brought me along carefully. (By the way, the five-pound restriction on women with lymphectomies has been debunked since my surgery.[4])

The other serendipitous event in my life that got me back into regular exercise was fundraising for Hope Connections. When Hope Connections had been affiliated with The Wellness Community, we had joined their fundraising program of "destination marathons," and several of our board members had participated. You know the routine: You agree to raise a minimum amount for a charitable organization, and the organization in exchange provides training to run a marathon as well as getting you to the event, putting you up, and so on.

I regretted not participating in one, despite my good excuse. Also, I am emphatically not a runner. The only running I had ever done was an occasional mile, and I mean one mile, in a vain attempt to take up running, but that faded immediately every time. John was a fairly regular runner, and I envied people who were. It seemed so simple with no need to go anywhere special or have much in the way of special equipment, and people who ran always looked so healthy and fit. Besides, I like being outdoors. So as I started to feel better in the fall of 2007, and as our CEO continued to push us as board members to raise money, I started to toy with the idea of joining in.

---

4 "Lymphedema and Exercise," www.breastcancer.org/treatment/lymphedema/exercise, October 9, 2019.

The next planned event was California's Big Sur marathon, but it had several shorter components, including a 10.6-mile race that covered the last 10.6 miles of the marathon course, all along State Route 1 on the Pacific Coast. I knew I wasn't going to be able to do a full marathon, but 10.6 miles sounded like something I could build up to with training. I didn't want to do it by myself, though. I figured John would be game for something that provided an incentive to run for both himself and me. Even Emma joined us. Running up the Pacific Coast sounded pretty amazing, so she said she was in.

Thus in January 2008 we met up with a group in Dupont Circle in Washington, D.C., with a trainer, Jeff Horowitz. Our group had a mix of ages, some in their twenties who had had a parent or other relative with cancer, and many in our forties, fifties, and sixties who were touched by cancer in some way. Emma, at age 11, was the mascot. We had a weekly run on Saturday mornings on some clever route Jeff developed around Washington, different and longer every weekend, and we were to run three to four other times during the week on our own, with those runs starting at two miles and going up for our group to six or so miles in the last few weeks. Training was hard—not only the actual running but also just showing up. It was a huge time commitment and required great discipline, particularly as we were in the dead of winter. The sky was dark until 7:00 a.m. and again after 5:00 p.m., but we had to run. We bought lights and reflective vests, hats and gloves, cool running jackets, and Sports Beans to keep us going on the longer runs. Emma gamely joined us on every run. I won't say she never complained. We all complained. We developed a game of naming a part of our body that didn't hurt: our teeth, our fingernails, our eyelashes.

I learned to run distances and really felt I had accomplished something. Not only that, we raised more than $20,000. It was incredibly heartwarming when we learned how many people had wanted to do something for us during my treatment but had been unable to because of distance or other circumstances. They gave generous amounts to a Washington, D.C., cancer support organization just because we asked. The actual event in April 2008 was taxing and tiring, and all three of us weren't sure we were going to make it. My sister Lucy flew out from New Jersey to support us in person, and we knew we had to cross that finish line for her and all the others who had donated on our behalf. We wore on our shirts the names of friends and family who had had cancer, some of them still alive, like my mother, and some not, like John's mother and Holly. They were an inspiration to us and made us accountable. The next day we couldn't walk or descend stairs, but that's a different story. It was a magical weekend in many ways because of the setting, because of the accomplishment, and because of the group we had trained with for four months and experienced the event with, all of them with a cancer connection.

There was another aspect of recovery that took me by surprise, and that was the odd experience of a kind of competition among breast cancer patients. All cancers exist on a spectrum—from manageable and not particularly dangerous to life-threatening. Mine was closer to the scary end of the spectrum. A friend e-mailed me recently seeking my and John's advice (an almost weekly occurrence for us), as her sister-in-law had just been diagnosed with triple-negative breast cancer. My friend "informed" me that only 10 to 20 percent of breast cancer is triple-negative, but that this type of cancer is very aggressive, so the doctors were recommending chemotherapy before surgery. She has known me for almost thirty years, and I wanted to scream: "I had triple-negative breast cancer! How did you not know that? Do you not know how lucky I am not to have had a recurrence? Do you know how scary it was?" I dropped the fact into my reply casually, and she replied, "I didn't know you had triple-negative."

I was hurt that people seemed not to realize that my odds were not good. The year I was undergoing treatment, my son came home and said a classmate was crying because her mother had breast cancer. It turned out she had DCIS, ductal carcinoma in situ. Since then, the assessment is that this is no longer considered cancer and that it should be a "watch and wait" situation. Even at the time, I wanted to say, "That's not *real* breast cancer. I am the one in actual mortal danger here."

Why did I feel this way? Why did I need to win this cancer competition? I was well aware that there were people with much worse cancers than mine, some who had metastasized, and some who had died, so I wasn't winning anyway (fortunately). But something about being in a life-threatening position brings out the worst in some of us. We need to have the fragility of our hold on life acknowledged and appreciated.

I also found competition about treatment and medical professionals. Who is treating you? What treatment are you having? Well, I'm going to the world-class Georgetown Hospital, where they specialize in breast cancer and have brilliant and kind staff, and I'm on three, count 'em, three, clinical trials. Of course, I never said anything like that. I felt competitive on the inside, but I had no desire to undermine anyone else's confidence in her own medical care. I didn't appreciate it when people questioned the care I was receiving. I had spent too much time trying to defend why I hadn't had immediate reconstruction to go down that path with someone else. I tried not to rise to the bait when other people seemed to want to pick a fight about who was getting the best care. All we want is for our healthcare team to know what they are doing and how best to treat our cancer. There is so little certainty, thanks in part to a new study in breast cancer making headlines each month, each study seeming to lead to a slightly different conclusion. We do need good, smart medical professionals to help us interpret and choose, and we need our healthcare system to ensure access to these talented medical professionals for everyone with a cancer diagnosis.

CHAPTER 27

Metastases or Hypochondria?

As part of my regular follow-up, I was to see Dr. Liu every six months and have a CT scan to see if any cancer or "suspicious spot" was visible in any part of my body or if that spot on my lung that showed up in the first CT had changed. I hated that scan. Naturally, I was glad someone was watching over me, but a CT scan was a little too deep a look. I was happily going along, not thinking about having cancer or potentially having cancer, and then it would be time for my CT scan. A few days before, I would get nervous imagining that I *might* have cancer, and life might change dramatically again in the next few days. I would slink over to the hospital, check into radiology, and curl myself into a ball over my crossword in the waiting room, trying to ignore everyone around me. I would wait silently for my name to be called, chat with the tech as if I hadn't a care in the world, and be escorted to the changing area.

I would don a hospital gown, sit shivering in the changing area as I waited, put on my brave and cheerful face for the CT scan operator, and lie still and follow instructions about breathing in and holding it while the machine loudly whirred around me. Then I would spend the rest of the day until Dr. Liu called trying not to think about what the scan might show and whether bad news was going to change the rest of my life. It was impossible not to think about it. Fortunately, it was always good news, but in a way, I could say that the scans retraumatized me. The relief of knowing that there wasn't any sign of cancer in my body was enormous, but the price felt high and sometimes unbearable. I would share my fears with John as the scan approached, and John seemed to find this particular anxiety less disconcerting. Maybe the scans actually scared him less than the chemotherapy or the cancer itself, so it was easier for him to talk naturally and sincerely about how I felt rather than responding with reticence.

In fact, he said he found that many of his patients are, in a weird way, relieved when they hear their cancer has metastasized because they have lived in constant fear of the "other shoe dropping," and now it has, so they can move on. I could understand that; there was a sort of bizarre desire to have the CT scan find cancer so I could check that box off. Obviously, should that occur, who wouldn't want to return to the cancer-free days? And yet the feeling illogically persisted.

Somehow, during the past year of treatment, John and I had seen a change in our relationship. While in many ways we had to work *more* as a team, and we each had to incorporate even *more* into our jampacked lives, we had begun to find our way back to each other as loving partners rather than just team members. Some of it came from the newfound time in doctor's offices and hospital rooms to be alone together. It's not the way we would have chosen to spend that time, but it had its advantages. In addition, I learned *a lot* about John's work and the toll it took on him. Cancer reminded me every day how lucky I was still to be on earth with someone whom I loved and who loved me.

I assume almost every current or former cancer patient is acutely aware of every change in his or her body and is hypervigilant. The downside of this, aside from generalized fear and anxiety, is that everything you find leads to more diagnostic tests. In March 2008, I had my routine semi-annual CT scan of my thorax and abdomen to check for metastases. Dr. Liu called me afterward to tell me the radiologist had seen a nodule on my ovary. She recommended that I have a vaginal ultrasound exam to be sure. Because of my relatively young age and aggressive breast cancer, I was at risk for ovarian cancer, so a few weeks later I went to the Georgetown radiology department for the vaginal ultrasound. The cyst had disappeared, but during those few weeks, I could feel the dread of an ovarian cancer diagnosis invade my days.

One year after I had finished chemotherapy, I was out for a run one day, and as I stopped to wait for cars to go by, I rubbed my fingers over the front of my left thigh. I was surprised to feel a fairly prominent lump on top of the quadricep muscle. I had never noticed it before, but my legs were more muscular from running, so perhaps it had been there all along and was just now noticeable. I called Dr. Liu to tell her and ask what I should do, acknowledging with embarrassment that I was becoming a hypochondriac. I asked if breast cancer could even *metastasize* to the leg. She assured me that it would be highly unusual, but she wasn't going to take risks. Once a cancer patient, always a cancer patient. The ultrasound of my leg wasn't conclusive, so I had *another* MRI; that showed "two very subtle, round, adjacent foci of signal change within the subcutaneous fat at the area of the larger palpable abnormality." That wasn't conclusive either. Dr. Liu suggested that I could have a needle biopsy of the area, which was probably the only test that might show anything now. She didn't seem to think it was necessary as she was fairly certain that the bump was some minor abnormality in the fat of my leg. I debated whether to move on to the next step, but I knew I wouldn't rest until I had more information, so I signed up for the needle biopsy. This one was just a regular needle inserted into the lump and a syringe pulled up to extract tissue and fluid. No pain, no real invasion. The doctor who performed it acknowledged my concern and the strangeness of the lump, then found nothing other than fat cells. Hypochondria, not cancer.

My next freak-out occurred in February 2009, when I lifted a heavy jug of water onto an upper shelf, and something went out in my neck and left arm. I called Dr. Liu again and apologized for being a hypochondriac again, but this one really hurt, and I couldn't lift my left arm above my shoulder. John was out of town, so I suffered alone. I had an MRI that evening. I left Emma at home to do her homework, telling her what was going on, and I drove to Georgetown during rush hour, worrying all the while. I had had neck pain at the time of my original diagnosis, and I remembered how concerned everyone had been about the possibility of cancer in the bone at that time. The Elizabeth Edwards story and how her metastases had presented, with a sore and fractured rib, haunted me. I had had neck pain before, and it was just that: neck pain caused by use of my neck and not by breast cancer, so it was likely the same thing.

Dr. Liu called the next day with the news that I had a herniated disk in my neck, but no evidence of bone metastases, and she sent me to see an orthopedist. He sent me to physical therapy after a two-week course of anti-inflammatories and some rest, and I eventually returned to normal. A herniated disc is not hypochondria; fortunately, it's also not cancer.

In the fall of 2009, Dr. Liu informed me in a tentative tone that my insurance company no longer would pay for regular CT scans unless I developed a symptom that suggested a metastasis and therefore merited a scan. She assured me that if they found something on a CT scan before I actually developed a symptom, it would not make a difference in my probable outcome. It came as a bit of a relief. I wasn't thinking about cancer every day, but I was acutely aware of my body and every change in it. At that point, finding a metastasis early might give me a little longer, but it wasn't going to keep me from dying of breast cancer. *Not* having regular CT scans meant not being starkly reminded every six months that it was possible I *could* have metastases. Not seeing every suspicious spot meant not having every available test to figure out what it might be. It was clear that even without routine CT scans, I was going to have repeated diagnostic testing over the years to come.

Later that fall, inspired by our first running event, we resolved to try doing another, so we signed up for the Mardi Gras Marathon in New Orleans. My sister even joined us to run this one. It was going to be a half-marathon for us, a jump in ambition, but we knew we could do it. We began training again with Jeff and the group in late 2009, but about a month before the event, in early 2010, I developed a sharp pain in my left thigh. Even I didn't think it was a metastasis, but I went through my usual panicky memories and flashbacks as I entered the MRI machine. The radiologist pulled me into his office afterward to tell me what he'd found. He didn't really know what it was, but he was fairly confident that it wasn't bone metastases. Unfortunately, he and the orthopedist thought I had a stress fracture in my thigh, which had been caused by an unusual side effect of the Zometa, so I had to go off that drug trial. I had to stop training for the run, too, which was very disappointing. John, Emma, and Lucy went on to complete the New Orleans half-marathon while I cheered them on from the sidelines. I wasn't too distressed about going off the Zometa, however. I had had almost the whole treatment, and the threat of necrosis of the jaw still made me nervous, never mind this unusual stress fracture.

Going off the Zometa trial meant that I needed to give up my mediport. I had held on to it for two and a half years after treatment, going in every month to get it flushed, using it for every follow-up CT scan that required IV contrast, and even managing to get one of my routine colonoscopies done with the IV run through the port instead of a vein in my arm. I didn't want to lose it, but it made no sense to keep it anymore. In fact, I was just past the three-year mark, starting with the original diagnosis in November 2006, and this was the time period in which one would expect a triple-negative breast cancer to recur, so I was becoming a little hopeful that I might not actually need the port at all. John also suggested that I was being a bit of a diva in using it for every procedure in the hospital, as it required going to the oncology infusion unit. Other medical techs and nurses were trained only to put in IVs, and I was taking the infusion nurses' time and attention away from people who actually had cancer in order to keep myself from having to do something that I didn't like but wasn't serious.

I reluctantly called to make an appointment to have the port removed. It was going to be under light anesthesia again and would take about half a day. The removal was undramatic. My port was gone, and all that remained were a few scars and my tattoos.

On November 28, 2009, I celebrated three years of cancer-free survival. Soon after my diagnosis, we were told that the silver lining of triple-negative breast cancer was that the risk of metastases significantly declined at the three-year mark. I felt healthy, and I had made it. We didn't have another party, but John and I acknowledged the anniversary out loud to each other, and we let out a joint sigh of relief.

The next two years passed quickly, made even more hectic by our usual full-speed-ahead lives. Cancer moved further and further away in the rearview mirror. In November 2011, it had been five years, and I was still cancer-free Maybe this was really behind us. John and Lucy held a big party for my fiftieth birthday in March 2013 and invited all our local friends and family, as well as the medical team that had gotten me to that point. We danced the night away to celebrate my making it to the mid-century mark. My best friend from college even sneaked into town to surprise me! I knew how lucky I was, both medically and personally. I finally could move on.

Except it turned out that the aftereffects of my cancer diagnosis weren't happening only to me; John was just beginning to feel the aftereffects on him.

CHAPTER 28

The Last Breast

Reconstruction of Liza's left breast was all about restored aesthetics; removal of the right was all about reduced risks. I understand the motives completely. After all, in my line of work, my patients have undergone truly major surgery, with colons, stomachs, pancreases, parts of livers, and esophagi removed. Those are all organs that we don't see in the mirror, but once missing, they change lives dramatically and significantly. Try eating a meal with no stomach, with no reservoir to hold the meal. Try digesting that chicken, rice, and broccoli without a fully functioning pancreas. Without enough digestive juices produced to break down dinner, the undigested food races through your GI tract, forcing an urgent, incredibly foul-smelling bowel movement about forty-five minutes after each meal. Imagine living every day interrupted by eight to twelve urgent bowel movements.

Of course, some of my patients grow weary of all the planning, of all the discipline required just to keep living. The stress of their job is too much, and they quit or are fired. They struggle with personal relationships and become loners. They lose weight and grow weaker. Yes, we cure an increasing portion of our GI cancer patients, but we leave a big scar that never really heals. They need a lot of help, and while we do our best, we fall short. For my patients, there is rarely a reconstruction to consider.

So after all that, what's the big deal about a mastectomy? After nursing, breasts have essentially no physiologic function. In fact, all other mammals' breasts come and go as needed. There is the sex thing, but you have two breasts, and one should do the trick.

Balance matters. Clothes need to fit. A bathing suit should not provoke anxiety. Public appearance has a lot to do with quality of life. I get all this. For most of my career, the breast machine has dedicated enormous resources in research trials to save breasts and to prevent the need for mastectomies. We trade the removal of an entire breast for a lumpectomy, at the cost of five to six weeks of radiation. Sure, you keep your breast, but it now glows in the dark!

Famously, Nancy Reagan was shamed by the breast community when she opted for a mastectomy instead of lumpectomy and radiation. As reported in the *New York Times* in 1988, "Rose Kushner, the executive director of the Breast Cancer Advisory Center in Kensington, Md., went so far as to say that Mrs. Reagan's decision 'set us back 10 years.'" She was sixty-six years old, and she was the First Lady. Going back and forth to radiation would cost the country added expense just in providing her additional daily security. And the outcomes of mastectomy compared with lumpectomy and radiation were the same. But, somehow, her decision to have a mastectomy was perceived as a slap, a failure to embrace the progress, a missed opportunity to set an example for others. "I couldn't possibly lead the kind of life I lead, and keep the schedule that I do, having radiation or chemotherapy," she told newswoman Barbara Walters. "There'd be no way. Maybe if

I'd been twenty years old, hadn't been married, hadn't had children, I would feel completely differently. But for me it [mastectomy] was right."

The only president who had colon cancer while in office was Nancy's husband. Add Ronald Reagan to the long list of missed opportunities for us GI cancer advocates. His case was swept under the rug, hushed up in the name of personal privacy. I believe the country was not yet willing to talk about colons. His White House handlers might have been embarrassed that he had missed the symptoms, and as he was the oldest president at that time, the Reagans might not have wanted any signs of weakness. And yet, by minimizing his diagnosis, fewer people were screened and more people died.

Liza was not offered a choice of a lumpectomy and radiation, and any thought of reconstruction had to wait until an undefined amount of time had passed. No one was sure that after the radiation, her remaining skin could withstand the added pressure of an implant, or that a transplanted flap of muscle and skin would even heal.

Liza was not in any hurry to have more surgery. She got new bras that could hold a prosthesis (Thank you, Nordstrom!), and she adjusted her wardrobe so that the asymmetry was not too obvious. She had pockets sewn into her bathing suits to insert a prosthetic. She was settling in for the long haul with one breast. For me, this was just fine. I really did not want anyone to do anything else major to her. One breast was plenty.

In social settings, when the subject of your wife's breast cancer comes up, it is wild to watch all the eyes in the circle go straight to your wife's breasts. They try to be subtle, with a quick glance, maybe a second longer glance. Looking closely, it's apparent that one breast is a bit lower than the other. So many questions just hang in the air, but everyone is much too polite to ask them. Liza, being the sensitive and aware person that she is, just came out and told them. Mastectomy to the right, original equipment on the left. Once the ice was broken, the conversation and questions continued, digging deeper. "I could not even tell!" "You look great!" "Will you get reconstruction?"

By this time, the breast cancer community had pivoted from sparing breasts with less surgery to removing both of them to reduce any risk of a second cancer. Appropriately, the aggressive surgical strategy started with the BRCA patients, those with a high risk of breast cancers due to an inherited genetic risk. These people also can get ovarian cancer and pancreatic cancer. Add prostate cancer to the list for men with BRCA. Some women also get their ovaries and uterus removed. No one gets their pancreas or prostate removed just to lower the risk; the surgery would be both too dramatic and too life altering. But as this approach was becoming more routine, the attitude of "take-both-of-these-things-off-of-my-chest-before-they-kill-me" was spreading through the non-BRCA breast community as well.

This is *not* analogous to elective plastic surgery. To remove the risk of cancer, all of the breast has to come off. Even the skin has to go, as breast tissue hangs on underneath. No nipple or other tissue that retains a sexual connection is left behind. Yes, as part of the rebuild, artists can tattoo you a terrific set of nipples, or maybe two different ones to be exotic. However, those are only for the observer, whether it is the person in bed with you or the person looking back in the mirror. It does not do anything more than provide a reminder of what once was there.

Liza did not want the plastic surgery simply to rebuild her right side. While she was not happy with it, she dealt with the asymmetry amazingly well. She also did not want to have surgery before she was more certain that her cancer was not coming back. What she really wanted was to remove the left breast, especially when it was time to screen her remaining breast, and she remembered how screening had failed the first time. She did not want to get burned again. She did not want even a chance of having to endure more chemo, radiation, mediports, and drains—certainly not because of some stupid breast that she was not using anyway.

And yet *I* cared about that breast. If that one goes, then I will never again in my life have sex with a woman with a breast. That part of my love life will be gone forever. No one ever said, "Sex will be different." (At least no one ever said it to me.) But, of course, it would be, and for the first time in this whole ordeal of Liza's cancer, I felt myself slipping into emotional states that were not those of the model, concerned, and supportive husband. I was sad about it. You might even say that I was grieving.

But now comes the unruly emotional part that I'm a bit ashamed of: I was angry at not even being asked for my feelings on the subject. I couldn't say anything about it. All I could do was support Liza's decision. The breast was not mine, so I did not get a vote. Liza's double mastectomy was another loss I could blame on the damn breast cancer machine, and one I would have to keep to myself. Up to this point, I had freely incorporated Liza's breast cancer experience as material in my rants, lectures, and editorials. But not this. This was out of bounds, and I could not vent my feelings about this surgery with anyone. Even though I knew the odds of a second cancer were low, I had no right to talk her out of the surgery just so I would have a breast in my sex life. Sure, I understood her decision: Losing her remaining breast now would remove her risk of dying of breast cancer later. She was open in explaining her rationale and risk/benefit calculation. I am pretty sure she incorporated me and our relationship into her decision algorithm, but I never knew what value she used because she never asked me.

But Liza was determined. Maybe she just wanted to feel more normal. I know she was tired of the glancing looks, tired of dealing with a prosthesis, tired of not being able to swim normally, tired of not fitting into clothes properly. As for her normal breast, she wanted as little risk as possible of another cancer, even at the cost of the increased risk of plastic surgery. Then, in the most surreal experience I had, the surgeon suggested making Liza a "bit bigger" than before. If we were going to go to all this trouble, she might as well.

Excuse me? Did we not just say that this was going to be a tight fit, and now the plan is to shove something bigger in there? All this to remove the risk of a second cancer and restore lost balance? Inside, I could hear myself scream, "The breast cancer world is fucking insane."

Virtually all patients of mine would like their ostomy reversed. Sometimes it's possible, but only when everything else is settled, all the treatment is over, and there is little chance for the cancer to come back. We make patients go a long time, pooping into a bag under their shirts, before we agree to reverse the ostomy. We ignore, postpone, or even refuse their number one desire to switch back their fecal stream, also known as number two, to its original path, concluding that in our medical judgment, it is not worth the risk of the surgery.

Who are we to judge the importance of restored function? How can we measure the distress behind their request? Our jobs are to relieve suffering, yet we often fail to hear the cry for help. We fail to understand patients' priorities when all they are asking of us is the chance for restoring a life closer to normal. For many patients, restoration to a new normal is worth whatever the added costs.

I totally understood Liza's decision for reconstruction. Gradually my initial anger, my feelings of grief and loss, lessened. I was feeling less sorry for myself as I understood Liza's priorities more. At this point, I again recognized that it wasn't all about me, but I was about to return to the caregiver role and watch someone whack another body part off the woman I loved. I was still sad.

Reconstruction is not really the best description of what we do. There is no way to restore what was lost, certainly not the way it was before the cancer. No matter how masterful the medical team, we leave a mark and a deficit. Life will be different, and there will be a new normal. Instead of reconstruction, it would be more accurate to describe what we do as a renovation, a remodeling, maybe a teardown to build something new.

Liza needed to do the surgery. I needed to respect that and move on.

CHAPTER 29

Reconstruction

I had officially entered the world of follow-up: semi-annual visits with Dr. Liu and Dr. Willey, and a semi-annual mammogram and ultrasound on my remaining breast. Dr. Willey was clearly concerned that I might develop a new cancer in the left breast. Every time I saw her, she would ask me if I was thinking about reconstruction yet. I would hem and haw and say I wasn't really ready. Of course, I had thought of reconstruction, but another surgery and everything that went with it, including a recovery period, didn't appeal to me at all.

Then she would suggest that I might want to think about having my other breast removed because of the way the first cancer had presented itself. Even after we knew a cancer was there, it really didn't show up on an MRI, or a CT, or a mammogram, so she wasn't confident that we could catch another one in time. She worried that such an aggressive cancer in my breast at my age might happen again. I had had the recommended genetic testing, and it had not revealed inherited cancer genes. I also knew that not being able to identify a genetic component didn't mean it wasn't there.

Finally, in 2012, my resistance began to break down, and my mental strength to endure more surgery and recovery began to build. Dr. Willey's warnings and my own experience with breast cancer frightened me. Early on, I didn't think it could happen. I had had breast cancer, checked that box. God would never give someone who had had cancer *another* cancer. But I knew that wasn't true. People get different cancers, a breast here, a colon there. John had several patients over the years who had suffered from a GI cancer and then called him a few years later for a referral to a different oncologist for a new cancer. The possibility of a new cancer in my left breast, particularly with my risk factors, was higher than average. As the years passed, and Dr. Willey reminded me of those facts every six months, I started to think that maybe I was tempting fate by clinging to my left breast.

I examined the left breast every morning in the mirror to see if it looked any different. I also went back to doing routine self-exams on it every month, palpating it almost obsessively to see if I could feel any bump other than the fibroadenoma that was already there. I even tried to see if I could feel a change in the size or shape of the fibroadenoma, as if I could really tell. And the first cancer hadn't been palpable anyway, so who did I think I was fooling?

But this decision was different from my first mastectomy. The first one involved no decision at all; it had to come off to save my life. With this one, I was making a deliberate decision to remove a healthy breast that we did not know would ever *develop* a cancer. Was a second mastectomy the right thing to do? I could wait and see what happened. That was running a risk, certainly, but how big a risk was it really? The percentages were low that I would develop a new cancer in the left breast. I could get a new cancer anywhere, and I wasn't going to remove all the parts of my body to prevent dying from one, so why this?

Yet the chances still *were* higher for a cancer in my left breast than other parts of my body, as Dr. Willey pointed out. She noted that if I had the left breast removed because of a cancer, I probably would have to have the lymph nodes removed on that side as well, which meant that I couldn't have blood pressure taken on either arm or have an IV given or have blood taken from either arm. That would be extremely complicated. I couldn't imagine how I would manage labs and medical procedures going forward if both arms were out of commission, never mind if I needed chemotherapy again. I wasn't sure if these were risks I was willing to run.

I was getting tired of the prosthesis and not looking normal. Being flat on the right side affected everything I wore. No pretty bras, limited options on bathing suits. Strapless or "strappy" tops required the prosthesis that stuck to my skin, a remarkable invention that did make a difference in how I could dress and therefore how I felt about myself, but nevertheless, it was still a rounded pyramid of gel that adhered to my skin. Nothing low-cut, as I had cleavage on only one side. (Is it still cleavage if there's only one side?) It was hard to feel alluring in my lacy nightgowns when one side of my chest was completely flat.

In 2012, Emma had started driving, and Charlie was attending college, so I was less essential for the day-to-day functioning of the family. If I took myself out of commission for a few weeks, the effects on everyone would be a lot less. I told John what I was thinking, that I had had enough of worrying about a possible cancer in the left breast, that Dr. Willey seemed to feel strongly that I was running a risk by keeping the breast, and that I would like to look more normal across my front.

I asked what he thought. He repeated back to me all the reasons I had given him for having the second one removed. I knew he wouldn't argue with me, that he felt it was my breast and therefore my decision, no matter what regret he felt about having a wife with no real breasts and no real nipples. I probably would have been angry if he had argued. How can a spouse offer an opinion on something like this in a way that sounds reasonable? "I won't want to have sex with you anymore if you remove your last remaining breast to lower your fairly high risk of breast cancer." I am fortunate to be married to a loving, unselfish man who deeply understands the hard and personal decisions people have to make after a cancer diagnosis. I also think that perhaps he wasn't willing to run the risk of another cancer and what that would mean for all of us.

Thus, in late July, John and I revisited Dr. Spear, a plastic surgeon who specialized in breast reconstruction, specifically in complex reconstruction. It had been five years since we first met, and during that time, whenever Dr. Spear saw John at Georgetown, he would ask, "Is your wife ready? I'm ready whenever she is." Now I was, and he was impressed with what he termed the "modest" radiation changes and praised Dr. Grayson for keeping my skin in such good shape. The inconvenience of living with goopy calendula lotion constantly on me for two months had paid off, and an implant was still an option. I sent a silent (and later spoken) thank you to Dr. Grayson for her skill and her care. Dr. Spear reiterated that the chance of things "working out reasonably well" was about 70 percent to 80 percent. He was careful to make sure I understood that choosing an implant was still risky for me because my skin had been damaged. His preference would be to put new, healthy, non-radiated skin there from another part of my body to increase the chances of a successful outcome, but he was willing to try the implant, and it had a reasonable chance of succeeding.

He said he would use Natrelle shaped and silicone-filled breast implants—he found them to be the best for smaller breasts—and he gave one to me. It was cold and firm but also malleable. I had no idea what a breast implant should look or feel like, but if it was the one he liked, so be it.

Dr. Spear then advised me of the risks of the surgery, particularly with respect to my radiated skin. For the rest of my life, I would need to take an antibiotic before every dental cleaning and procedure. Sometimes bacteria can get in the bloodstream from dental work, and they like to travel to and make their home in foreign substances in the body, such as breast implants. He cautioned that my right breast might not heal properly because, as he put it, radiated skin didn't really see the point in putting out the effort to heal. It might do a superficial job and be more likely to get an infection. If that happened, he would have to go back in and remove the implant, and we would have to try something else. There was a risk the implants could leak at some point down the road, which would require their removal, simple but daunting. And there was a risk of "capsular contracture," in which fibrous tissue builds up around the implant and can cause the breast to become hard, stiff, and distorted on the chest. That also would require removal of the implant.

As for the surgery itself, I would need drains again, one on each side, both now and in about six months when Dr. Spear would go back in to replace the expanders with implants. I would have the risks of surgery generally—death under general anesthesia, infections, bleeding, and so on. I listened, but I wasn't going to see Dr. Spear and take up his time again if I wasn't ready to do this now. He also warned me that this surgery was going to be more painful for longer than the post-mastectomy period because the expanders had to be placed under my pectoral muscle, which would make it "unhappy" for a while, leading to spasms for three to four weeks after the first surgery.

I went through the picture-taking and the paperwork, and the office staff conferred with Dr. Willey to find a time both surgeons were available. She would remove the left breast before Dr. Spear stepped in to do his work. We settled on November 20, 2012, two days before Thanksgiving. Great, another Thanksgiving disrupted by my medical problems. I had to coordinate with Dr. John's schedule as well, and a holiday meant a few days when work wouldn't drag him away.

John and I probably had a small farewell party for the other breast; I don't remember. I'm sure we didn't invite any guests. But having already lost all sensation on the right side with the removal of that breast, I was going to have to accept losing sensation in my entire breast area, a part of intimacy I was going to miss. I was pleased that I was going to *look* whole again, even if I wasn't really going to *be* whole. I would not have nipples or even the appearance of nipples on either breast. I had decided against "nipple-sparing" surgery on the left side; I worried that any remaining breast tissue would increase my risk of getting another breast cancer. A nipple would have no sensation, and it just ran the risk of complicating the surgery and recovery.

One plus of breasts with implants is that they stay in position without support even as you age. I wasn't going to have to wear a bra if I didn't want to. I also would be able to wear a swimsuit without a prosthesis, and I wouldn't have to worry about sagging for many years.

On the morning of November 20, I returned to the Surgery Center at Georgetown Hospital in a much cheerier mood than the last time I had been there. Yes, I was nervous about surgery in general, but I was excited about the improvements that were to come in my daily life and my view of myself. While I hadn't been particularly distressed by the way I looked, and I was truly just grateful to be alive, my heart sang a bit now. Dr. Spear came by to see me and draw in Sharpie on my chest to be sure that we all agreed on what he was going to do and where he was going to do it. Then it was off to the operating room.

When I awoke, Dr. Willey told me that they would send my left breast to pathology to be sure there was no cancer in it, but the results wouldn't be back for several days. So there was no news to impart other than that the surgery had gone well and that I had a tissue expander on each side of my chest with 50 cc's of fluid in each. I spent a night in the hospital and went home the next day, back in my oversized button-front shirt with drains pinned to the inside of it. Fortunately, I still had many of the clothes I had purchased in 2006 for my first surgery, so I made good use of them again.

Thanksgiving 2012 was odd but memorable if only through a haze from all the drugs to manage the pain from my pectoral muscle's unhappiness at being fiddled with. I spent the whole day mostly sound asleep on our family room sofa. Charlie was away for Thanksgiving, so it was just the three of us. John, being the intrepid host and cook, insisted that we should have my parents and sister for Thanksgiving dinner; I managed to convince him to order a cooked turkey and side dishes at least. Blurrily, I remember that John and Emma seemed to be watching a variety of strange nature shows every time I woke up, and then my parents were there. I sat at the dining room table for about fifteen minutes and then declared that I was unable to stay upright, so I returned to my supine position on the family room sofa.

The surgery was more extensive than my first mastectomy, which meant that this recovery was slower. I remained on pain and anti-spasmodic medication for about three weeks, as the pectoral muscle continued to spasm, but it finally relented. Then I spent the next few months having my expanders periodically injected with another 50 cc's of saline to expand them and the skin that overlay them—a strange but not painful experience. Once I had the expanders in, I asked Dr. Spear if we could make my breasts a bit larger than they had been. He, of course, was unfazed by this question but reminded me that we would be limited by the elasticity or lack thereof of the skin of my right breast. In the end, he was able to expand my right breast (and left as well, but there was no issue there) to a B cup, so I was pleased.

My April 2013 surgery to replace the expanders with implants was outpatient, and at this point, it was clear that John was done with my medical problems. He checked me in and went to work. Getting him to pick me up to take me home was a different matter. The nurses had gotten me settled where outpatients wait to go home once they are deemed sufficiently conscious and functional, and I had some juice and crackers. Someone had called John to tell him I was done and ready, but he didn't appear. I called him, and he said he'd be by in a bit to get me. Minutes and then hours passed, and the nurses asked me what was going on and why I was still there. Was my husband ever going to pick me up? I laughed wryly and said he'd come when he was ready. Clearly, I had moved back down his list. I chafed at being left in the outpatient waiting area for several hours, but I recognized that the fact we both could be blasé about this surgery was a good sign. We were almost done with breast cancer.

We were so blasé, in fact, that three days after the surgery, we drove to Durham, North Carolina, for John's thirtieth college reunion—me with drains in both sides of my chest and bandaging on my breast area.

Packed in our luggage were cups to empty the drains into and the chart to note the twice-daily drain output. We were old hands at this by now.

Duke University has always been a happy place for us, so we were regular class reunion attendees to catch up with our friends and to reminisce as we walked the campus. We weren't going to miss this year if we could avoid it. Dr. Spear had given us the go-ahead, and we took it. I didn't look so hot with my Michelin man appearance from the surgery bra and drains hidden beneath yet another oversized button-front shirt, but I was with friends who all knew what we had been through, so they greeted us joyfully and hugged me gingerly, being careful not to squeeze.

My breasts healed well, and I was delighted with my new appearance. This surgery was an easy one to come back from; the hard part had been done during the expander phase. I now had two same-sized breasts, or at least breast-like appendages in the correct place on my chest, which were going to make me look pretty much like a normal person again.

But as I healed, I began to notice that John's behavior and mood seemed to be changing. He was moving away from his normal.

CHAPTER 30

John's Turn

As 2013 progressed, I started to feel as if the "whole breast cancer thing" was behind me. My old, scary breasts were gone, and in their places were new breasts that didn't even need a bra. My chances of a recurrence were so low as to be insignificant compared with all the other risks in anyone's life. I felt healthy and was getting fit again, thanks to my trainer, who had adjusted my training at each step of the way to accommodate my various surgeries as well as the quotidian aches and pains of middle age. And I had become middle-aged! Hurray!

John was middle-aged, too, but he didn't seem to be as grateful as I was. He began talking of midlife crises, questioning what he was doing at work and why he was doing so much of it. His patients seemed to be taking a real toll on him. After my diagnosis, John started giving out his personal e-mail address to his patients. I didn't think it was a great idea, but I admired his generosity and deep desire to make life better for everyone going through cancer treatment. The day we received my diagnosis from Dr. Willey and met with her to come up with a treatment plan, John, appreciating the swift and smooth sched-uling of everything that had to happen thanks to our "insider" status at Georgetown, emphatically declared to her, "We've got to figure out a way to make this happen for every patient at Lombardi!" She seemed taken aback, hesitated a second, and then responded, "Yes, wouldn't that be great?" John apparently decided then and there that he was going to do what *he* could to replicate the kind of care I received and give every patient "the insider experience" at Lombardi.

In the beginning, it wasn't too bad. Patients were respectful, cautious, and grateful. They e-mailed only when it seemed absolutely necessary. Of course, with people being people, and cancer patients being in almost constant fear for their lives, and Washingtonians being used to getting what they want when they want it, patients started to become more blasé about their e-mail communications with their medical oncologist. When John gave his e-mail address to a patient and his or her caregiver, he would instruct them when it was all right to use it and when they should communicate with their care team through other avenues. He emphasized that he frequently didn't check e-mails on weekends or in the evenings, so they should not send urgent questions at those times. (That wasn't really true; he checked his e-mail frequently in the evenings and on the weekends.) I could see his exhaustion increase when he got one from a patient during his time away from work. One Sunday afternoon, after a day that included church and household chores, John wandered into the family room, sank into a chair, and opened his laptop. I heard him moan and then wryly laugh. "What?" I asked. He sighed. "A patient sent me an e-mail Friday night that describes a medical issue he was having and ends, 'I think I might be dying.'"

"What are you going to do?" John laughed again. "I responded, 'Did you die?'"

I laughed, too, at the patient's effrontery in assuming that John constantly checked his e-mail in real time to help this particular patient who thought he might be dying on a Friday evening, and who had a whole care team available then for just that purpose. I also laughed at John's cheeky response. Still, I could feel my heart sink as I watched John deal with this intrusion on his weekend and the expectation that he is always on call, always available. (For the record, the patient did not die that weekend nor soon thereafter, and he had the good grace to be chastened by John's response.)

It's a funny story, and John, with his usual good humor and loving attitude toward his patients, managed to handle it in a way that conveyed his point while not alienating someone who was scared and suffering. However, it is also an example of the personal cost of giving patients such access. He had at least one patient and probably more who would call his cellphone every time she had a question, no matter the time. She had gotten his cell number when he once called her from it, but he had not told her she could contact him that way. This did not stand in her way since she considered her questions far more important than his need for a personal life and some downtime from an extremely demanding line of work.

As the years passed, even John's most respectful and apprecia-tive patients began to step over the line and to take advantage of his openness and warmth, confusing it with constant availability for their needs. They would forget to ask for prescriptions when they were in the office and would e-mail him two hours later to say they needed him to call in their local pharmacy, forcing him to stop what-ever he was doing and return to their file to complete the task. As the frequency of these contacts increased, I could see John grow ever more tired and frustrated. He said he felt like a service provider who was expected to be available to all his patients for whatever they wanted, whenever they wanted it. The result was that he was losing some of the love he once had for the practice of medicine.

Meanwhile, his clinic was starting to fill with younger patients suffering extremely bad cancers. He had to talk to parents who were facing not seeing their young children grow up and others who were facing being a single parent. He knew what that felt like, and he knew what it felt like to lose a parent to cancer. He carried their burdens with him almost all the time, frustrated that he couldn't provide a cure, angry at the lack of progress in the treatment of GI cancers. He railed publicly about seeing young people in this situation, trying to egg on research into why so many young people were getting GI cancers.

And he got really tired.

John's travel also increased as he received more invitations to speak to doctors or consult on new drugs. Almost every day, he fended off invitations to speak all over the country and all over the world. The constant need to figure out what he could do and when he had to say "no" to myriad people asking for his time and energy was wearing him down. As chief of the division of hematology and oncology, he was the administrative head of a large group of doctors, nurses, case managers, and a complex staff of healthcare providers. Anyone who has ever managed people knows how much the issues, large and small, can take out of the person who is expected to resolve them.

When I first met John, he was a charmer and the class clown. That's a lot of what attracted me to him. He cared about what he did, and he wanted to make a mark in the world, but he didn't take anything too seriously. He was an iconoclast who poked holes in any balloon filled with hot air. Yet somehow he did it in a way that frequently made the person at the center of his joke laugh at his or her own folly. Now he had, as one of his co-workers told him, "lost his sparkle." He looked haggard. Most important, he seemed to have lost his ability to brush things off, to respond to the vagaries of life with humor. He was making *me* look like the funny, easygoing one, and that was not my role in this marriage.

A few years after my final surgery, we attended a Georgetown University basketball game at the downtown arena in Washington. As with all large crowd events, the security detail on the way in repeatedly barked rapid-fire commands to unzip your coat, put your cellphone in the basket, and remove all metal from your pockets, followed by a trip through the metal detector. On this Saturday afternoon, John for some reason kept setting the metal detector off, and the security officer kept ordering him to check his pockets again and go back through. After the second attempt, John began ripping off his coat and his belt, and he rather violently threw them on the table and berated the security guard. I was shocked. I rarely had seen John get so angry, and never about something so trivial. It was as if he had reached a breaking point of one more person telling him to do things that he just couldn't handle. He finally made it through, and after we collected our belongings, and he calmed down, I asked if he was OK. "I've never seen you like that," I said. He seemed ashamed of his strong response and apologized, but an apology was not what I felt was necessary at all. "I'm just worried about you," I said.

When we got home, Emma, who was back from college that weekend, was sitting at the kitchen table, watching something on her computer, and eating a snack. After John passed through the room, I described what had happened, and she too said she noticed that her father was becoming more sensitive. She wondered what had happened to his sense of humor. We had each gone to therapy over the years to deal with issues that were causing us emotional distress, and we had found it beneficial. Maybe this would be good for John, the man who was everyone's confidant, the non-board-certified psychiatrist for patients who were suffering emotionally. His stress, and yes, his depression, though we would never call it that, were the last severe side effects of my cancer diagnosis.

As we were putting dinner together that evening, Emma started the conversation. She said she had noticed that he seemed stressed recently. John tried to shrug it off and looked reproachfully at me for sharing what happened at the game. I seconded what Emma said, and slowly, gently, we got to the point of suggesting that he might find it beneficial to do a little therapy as well. He stopped being defensive and seemed almost grateful for the "intervention." "Yeah," he said, "that would probably be a good idea."

I have no idea what went on during those weekly sessions. But slowly and subtly, something seemed to shift. I could see that he was beginning to imagine his life differently. He was planning for a future that was not just clinical care and frantic travel. For the first time in his life, he talked about taking a sabbatical.

CHAPTER 31

Caregiver 2.0

Initially, intractable insomnia was *my* worst side effect from all of this, but in reality, the most dramatic, life-changing side effect I got from Liza's cancer was on my ability to do my job. Having lived the experience, having walked the walk, I felt that I was given a unique vantage point. I now saw our world of cancer care from both sides, consumer and provider. Right after Liza's cancer, I was inspired and energized to use my newly enlightened awareness for good, to help as many patients as I could. I was going to be the best doctor I could, using my experience and my position to ease the burdens of my patients and their caregivers.

I am not sure how soon after Liza's diagnosis this started, but with almost every new patient I saw, I shared our experience and made it personal, intimate. I ended our hour-long visits by pointing at the patient and saying, "My wife sat there." Then I pointed at the spouse and said, "And I sat there." I wanted them to know that I knew what it felt like "over there." I would riff on what it was like for us, how Liza's diagnosis impacted our lives, our kids, and our village. Delivered with a pointed finger, I would say that it was *the caregiver's* diagnosis, too, and that often the caregiver's role can be tougher than the patient's. I wanted them to begin their journey with the insights I had learned the hard way as well as the awareness I had wished for during our journey.

Was my sharing our story a cheap, sideshow trick? Did I turn what they were going through into something about me? Or did I offer a truly useful demonstration of support and understanding? Maybe it was unfair and misleading to share our story, the one that ends with Liza's survival—particularly with patients I knew were going to die. I wanted to be personal as a way to help ease the pain in front of me. What never occurred to me was that this would cost *me* in the end. I had so much to give, I could ease suffering, and I had developed a superpower.

For several years, I felt as if our efforts were having a real impact. We established new positions on our team to provide a one-phone-call entry point for all new patients. We worked more closely with our nursing teams to learn from each other, improving the cancer patient's and caregiver's experiences. We worked to improve the clinic flow so that patients' time would be spent more efficiently. I also preached my new gospel to our doctors, especially to our training doctors, so that they could be among the converted. I became evangelical about this in my lectures and writings. I used my new insights to shape the fundamental principles of our GI cancer research center, emphasizing a strategy with care based on the simple premise: how I would want to be treated when it was my turn.

On the research front, I became less excited by large, randomized trials that were designed to make only small gains, favoring instead smaller phase I and phase II trials that were designed to look for "home runs." I wanted to invest in high-risk, high-return research. We should be in more of a hurry to cure cancer. I could not understand why there was no sense of panic among the research and advocacy communities. People are dying, for God's sake, dying every day of these common, dreadful diseases. We are spending huge amounts of money, but we are not spending it wisely. I felt like Don Quixote, tilting at windmills, or John the Baptist, running around with a critical message of salvation.

I am not sure when, but it got harder. I still had the vision, I knew what we needed to maintain and how to evolve as a cancer center, but should I be the one to lead the next charge? Maybe my time at the top was over, best left to a new vision and fresh energy? Maybe my vision was simply unachievable. My batteries were taking longer to recharge. I felt as if a *Harry Potter* dementor was lurking and sucking all the goodwill from my soul.

It took more than ten years. I accumulated wear and tear, the added emotional burden with every new patient and caregiver with whom I shared Liza's and my stories, every patient who died, every teenage child I met with to explain what was happening to their parent, every bad scan, every tearful discussion—another month, another season, another year. I was getting worn out.

As my energy was being depleted, I found myself losing hope and faith. Maybe most unsettling was a growing sense of apathy. How could a doctor who was as committed as I had been become apathetic to curing cancer and caring for the sick? I was wondering how many more years I could do this. Would I ever achieve my goals and see my vision become a reality? And if not, why bother? It was becoming clear that I could never replicate Liza's amazing cancer care for every patient we treated. Why put myself through all of this extra work, the life-shortening stress, the precious time away from family if we are all going to die anyway? The cancer machine will keep on churning out products and making advances whether I am part of it or not. I am only a small part of a multi-billion-dollar global effort, with little chance for disruption from me alone. Maybe I need to rethink things. Maybe God had not called me to do this. Maybe I had misheard what I thought God had said.

Is this what burnout feels like? No. I'm much too strong to burn out, I told myself. Burnout is something that happens to the weak and the unloved. If I could burn out, then everyone must be burning out. But why aren't they saying anything to me? I am their chief, their mentor, and their friend. I assumed that they would come to me if they were feeling this way, too. Maybe it was just me.

I needed to change something, or I would break. For the next few years, I took on new roles that would give me a fresh focus and hopefully new energy. Instead of worrying about our local center and the patients in our region, I decided to go global. Now that would be disruptive! Current estimates show only one in seven people on our planet has access to cancer care as we know it; mostly it's just too expensive. Let's joust at that windmill for a while. Maybe that will recharge my batteries! My bosses were supportive, allowing me to reduce some of my local duties to dedicate more time externally, building first a U.S.-based and now a global alliance to expand access to cancer care. Forget trying to provide concierge-level care for everyone in D.C.—let's try to get *some* care to parts of the world where there is none.

The work was exciting, and it did recharge my batteries. But I was still feeling the weight of my patients. It seemed that each week we would lose one, only to be replaced by another, with a new story and new pain that needed to be lessened. I love caring for patients and their families. But if all I do with my calling is see one patient at a time, delivering today's standard of care, I will fall short of my potential. I must do all I can to have an impact on cancer outcomes, and that means disrupting the status quo. There has to be some reason for my mother's death, some reason for Liza's breast cancer and her survival. Just like my dad, I had big ideas. I needed time, maybe one last chance, to see them through.

Sabbaticals are a rarity among academic physicians. Sure, the entire French department takes off every seven years, but no Georgetown physician had taken a sabbatical in more than twenty years. Leaving work for six to twelve months is different for us clinicians. Yes, the French department faculty have to find someone to teach their classes for the semester, but I have to abandon my patients and my colleagues, asking them to pick up the slack while I am away. It was increasingly evident that I needed the break. Because...I needed it to do the global work. Besides, Liza and I also needed it to write this book. Writing our story has become the therapy I have needed all along: care for the caregiver. Maybe for once I would take the advice I so regularly have handed out: "Don't forget to live."

The six months leading up to my sabbatical was possibly the most stressful time of my life. I needed formal approval from the leadership at Georgetown, plus support from my colleagues and my patients. My blood pressure rose, requiring additional meds and cardiac stress testing. Despite the negative test, I continued with chest pain. Certain I was dying of an aortic dissection, I went to the ER on a Sunday night for what turned out to be my every-five-year emergency CT scan (likely true of all oncologists). Fortunately, it ruled out both my hysterical dissection and lurking cancer. Insomnia returned, and I was tough to be around at home. With just Liza and me there, instead of enjoying our empty nest, I was moody, short in my responses to even basic questions, with no interest in going to the theater or even to Nats games, my most sacred refuge from the real world. Looking back, I am sure that Liza was careful around me, hesitant to confront my behavior. She was under a lot of stress, too, managing her aging parents and my family members who needed her help, holding us all together while her world was just as unstable. The process of pushing the pause button on my job was killing me; if it didn't, I suspect Liza would have.

Most of the stress came from telling my patients. I knew that I was letting them down, breaking our unwritten contract. Liza kept saying that a sabbatical, where I would be returning after a year, was much better for the patients than my leaving Georgetown altogether, or worse still, really developing a medical problem. I still found it hard to meet with each of them in turn, wanting to tell them face-to-face before they received the official letter informing them of my plans. Almost without exception, the initial reaction included expressions of abandonment and panic, as if I had severed their few remaining strands of hope. But with few exceptions, the negative emotions quickly were followed by expressions of support, wishing me well. They too had seen the changes in me, and they worried about me and my condition. They bought into my big vision, wanting me to succeed in my global efforts. They understood the need for disruption, hoping that my efforts would help them or many others in the years ahead, those who do not yet know they will develop a GI cancer. I promised them that I would still be there for them, both in spirit and, if they really needed to reach out, by e-mail or phone.

Liza was the one who had cancer. She had the surgeries, the chemo, and the radiation. She was left with a new normal that includes neuropathy, reconstructed breasts, fear of lymphedema, and worry about second cancers. She has both visible and invisible scars from the cancer experience, but Liza rarely dwells on it. She has no pity parties. She made the entire process as easy on me and our family as she could.

Liza was thoughtful enough to get a serious disease with which I was intimately familiar. She was nice enough to get her care in my cancer center. She enrolled in clinical trials, and she added a platinum in response to a single e-mail, enduring more treatment than is standard. She rarely complained, even when things were rough. She downplayed her side effects so much that the kids and I have few memories of them. Liza mostly moved on from her personal journey with cancer, increasing her energy and focus on others as she doubled down on supporting other patients through Hope Connections. Liza was nice enough not to die.

Then why was it me who broke down in the end?

Even now, after I've reflected on my experience with Liza's cancer, I really do not remember many specifics about her actual treatments. I have no specific memory of how I felt or how the children reacted. Maybe I was too busy juggling my job and family to set down any memories. Maybe I was the one with chemo brain. I often explain chemo brain not as a chemical alteration in the brain from the drugs, but instead the human inability to keep up with all the added requirements and distractions that occur during cancer treatment. Many of us can juggle three balls, and I mean actually juggle three balls. But how about four, how about five? How about five balls and a chainsaw? (If I could do this, I would be touring with Cirque du Soleil.) I do remember juggling the three balls I had to keep in the air, but regularly dropping ball four, ball five, and the chainsaw, somehow keeping all my fingers and toes.

Liza's doctors taught me many new lessons. I learned that the time with the doctor was precious, and every minute, every second counted. Families and patients were always waiting for us, watching the clock, putting off lunch, risking the parking meter expiring, skipping the overdue trip to the grocery store, waiting for that one minute when the doc shows up to give the results and to provide the big picture. I became sensitive to the fact that our patients are watching for even the subtlest clues: our tone of voice, a glance at the watch, the raised eyebrow. We doctors are always on stage.

I remember going up to visit Liza while she was "being infused"—a terrible term in our oncology vocabulary, conjuring images as diverse as things done to tea leaves and to dead bodies. I would sit by her for a while, and sometimes we chatted and caught up. Sometimes she simply slept. Being terrible at just sitting with someone, I would not stay long and instead would scamper off to see a patient nearby or answer a page. I realized that a lot of cancer care ultimately is endured alone.

I knew what getting chemo was like. I understood that I was going to be asked to support Liza, give her shots at home, monitor her side effects, and attend clinic visits with her. I thought I was going to be so great at this caregiver stuff—who could be any better? In fact, I really had no idea of what was ahead and what Liza was about to go through. I knew how to *give* chemo; I had no idea what it was like to *get* it.

I remember that Liza was tired, and her fatigue was out of proportion to her blood counts or the known side effects of either the drugs or the radiation. She slept a lot, went to bed early, and napped often. I also remember that our lives went on pretty normally. We went out to plays, games, and dinners. We saw friends. Liza drove everywhere, often driving herself back and forth to chemo. We rarely missed church. Liza paid the bills (thank God), shopped for the groceries and the kids' clothes, and cooked many meals. We took few extra precautions to avoid infections, despite the nurses' warnings. She had no serious complications and only a few moderate ones. She never had to be admitted to the hospital, as so often happens as a consequence of this type of treatment. We were lucky; life went on.

I might not remember much because of some subconscious PTSD avoidance strategy. But maybe there was not much to remember.

As Liza progressed through treatment, the wear and tear certainly became more prominent, a greater burden for her and for me. But cycle by cycle, week by week, landmark moment by landmark moment, we both gained confidence. I have forever given patients advice that was in danger of being a cliché. "Once you get started, once there is a plan, once a few cycles of treatment are under your belt," I would say, "it gets easier." Who could have predicted that this was actually true?! We felt some earth beneath our feet, finally landing after a long free fall.

We could plan again, not very far in the future, but we could plan. Liza was not going to die today. She was not likely to die tomorrow. We remembered Holly, how quickly her cancer roared back, and how suddenly it killed her. I remember many of my patients with similar courses, here one day, gone the next. With every negative test, every day without cancer, we were closer to getting out of this. We were vigilant, looking for signs of its recurrence. We hate surprises. Nothing was going to sneak up on us again.

Life would be so much easier if we knew the date and time of our death. Think how easy big decisions would be. We would know how much money to save and when to buy that Tesla. We would know when to say our good-byes, and we would dramatically reduce our health-care expenditures—maybe even stop flossing our teeth. Our Google calendars would have an end date beyond which we couldn't schedule anything. I apparently have a meeting in 2078 on a Tuesday—I just checked. I will be one hundred seventeen years old. Maybe I will call in instead.

The Washington Post ran a story about a woman who was celebrating the end of her breast cancer treatment. She and a bunch of friends were on a beach in California when a rockslide fell on them, killing her and some friends. She had just endured the most destabilizing time in her life and made decisions about surgery, chemo, maybe radiation, and reconstruction. She sacrificed her long-term well-being, endured treatment-related side effects, gave up some of her "quality time" for even a 3 percent increased chance of being cured. She did this in the hopes of living longer—only to be dumped on and smothered, buried alive by a wrathful, mocking god. Was she being punished for celebrating? Was God actually sparing her from some future trauma by taking her suddenly now? Maybe God was really aiming at her friends, and she was just in the wrong place at the wrong time.

After finishing the article, I looked up from the paper at Liza cleaning up the morning dishes. She hadn't died from her breast cancer when the odds were that she certainly could have. She had not died in a car crash; no large rock had fallen on her from above. Life is already random enough, and cancer only makes this worse. I read her the story aloud, and we both laughed. We were not laughing at the unfortunate woman, not laughing at the breast cancer machine that could not prevent this one patient from dying. Our smiles arose from our feeling very lucky and blessed to still be alive and to still be together. Life throws stuff at us all, and we do our best to weather the storms, to duck out of the way, driven to survive for one more day, what we saw as another bonus day to share with those around us. We laughed at being lucky enough to have yet one more bonus day.

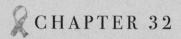

CHAPTER 32

The Kids Are All Right...Right?

John and Liza, as they did with their actual children,
created this chapter jointly.

harlie and Emma were born into a cancer family, a TV stuck
on the *Cancer Channel*. We have talked a lot about cancer all
their lives: the cancer experience of each of our mother's, the
almost weekly discussions we have about some friend, or friend of a
friend, who asked us to help navigate cancer. They knew that people
died from cancer. Over dinner, John often shared a story from clinic
that day, or about some family he met on rounds, or one of his partner's
cases that had reached him due to some issue, complaint, or doctor-patient tension interfering with the delivery of optimum care. Charlie
and Emma have been hearing these stories since birth, maybe from in
utero. (Most parents play music to the fetus; we talked cancer.) Given
the amount of medical information that flows around our house, the
whole family is well trained on all points HIPAA.

It's easy to know the kind of day John had. Sometimes it's been a
hard day at the office. He comes home tired and subdued after telling
people they are going to die, or watching someone die, or dealing with
a family's unrealistic goals of care, or having a day with one too many

bad scans. Then there are the good days. He's funny, energetic, maybe even ebullient when he walks in the door. Maybe he "graduated" a patient to five-year-time-for-a-big-party-no-need-to-see-me-anymore status, obtained a grant, gave a chalkboard talk to the fellows on colon cancer, or had a team member publish a paper in the *New England Journal of Medicine*. Maybe it's as simple as having a string of patients where cancer was shrinking.

Charlie and Emma lived through the Holly saga, too. Charlie and Holly's daughter were classmates, and the Richardsons were friends of ours. But they lived it even more because we didn't protect them from what we knew about what was going on with Holly. We didn't make a point of talking to them about it, but we also didn't take our discussions behind closed doors. Even at their age, they knew those conversations stayed in the house, not to be shared on the playground or anywhere else.

John also involved the kids in his work even more directly. In the spirit of "Take Your Kid to Work Day," Charlie and Emma often found themselves on rounds some weekend mornings, serving as sort of "therapy kids" for John's patients. On occasion, they ended up in the back of a classroom or lecture hall where John was giving a talk. Sometimes John would take them on his business trips, which both he and the kids loved. He wanted them to understand the tradeoffs of life, the reasons why he was not at every baseball game or all too often missed dinner at home or breakfast before school. Career versus family. But of course, like every proud parent, he also wanted to show them off. He wanted his world to meet the creator of Emma's room. He wanted them to meet his amazing son who could drive a golf ball 250 yards at the age of twelve.

Our family's approach to cancer as a dinner table topic and as a part of the family history even before Liza got cancer was to joke about it. "Yeah, well, my mother's DEAD!" John would say. "What's wrong this time?" Liza would ask. "Someone has cancer again?" Humor gave us all a vehicle to talk about what was happening while keeping it at a distance. Once Liza got cancer, we joked that we were *really* "the cancer family—all cancer, all the time." Liza's cancer was framed as yet another sacrifice for John's career so he could learn about it from the *inside*. He could have a "secret shopper" at George-town who could tell him how things really ran for those on the other side of the examining table. Liza wasn't afraid to play the cancer card at home. It was better to bring it into the open, to treat it as a normal part of our life as it was then. One night as Liza was starting to do the dishes, she suddenly felt exhausted. The kids were in the family room watching an episode of *SpongeBob* for the hundredth time. "Hey, kids, I don't feel like doing the dishes tonight. I have cancer, you know." They did not spring up and run into the kitchen; they didn't even look up. John took over the dishwashing.

When Liza was diagnosed, we carefully planned what we were going to say to them. We figured they had no idea there was anything wrong. Actually, Emma remembers hearing us say something in our bedroom a few days earlier about Liza's breast, but being Emma, she wanted no part of this discussion. And Emma saw John at school the day we got the diagnosis, and she instantly knew that something was wrong.

We thought we told Charlie and Emma everything that night and thereafter. We thought we were balanced, age appropriate, and trans-parent. Charlie was thirteen, and Emma was ten. They had few ques-tions, if any; they were both cancer savvy already. Stay tuned: Next on the *Cancer Channel* at 8 o'clock, *Your Mother Has Breast Cancer*; at 9, *Fun with Colonoscopies.*

They took part in wig shopping, and Liza made both the kids see her bare-chested a few weeks after the surgery, telling them that they were going to have to see it when she was old, and they had to take care of her, and she wanted them to be prepared. Charlie joined Liza in the infusion unit one day when she was having her port flushed, sitting in a small room with two other patients and their caregivers. He seemed to take it all in stride, cheerfully chatting with the roommates. Curing Liza of cancer was a family affair.

At school, both Charlie and Emma received lots of support. Charlie's classmates, already having experienced Holly's struggle with breast cancer, wrote a lovely card for Liza, which each one of them signed with words of encouragement. One of Charlie's classmates, to our surprise, used Liza and her breast cancer as a point in the annual eighth-grade speech competition, with the families of all the eighth-graders listening raptly. Was Charlie proud or uncomfortable?

Emma's experience of support in the school community was a bit different. She says now that she resented everyone treating her as if she was fragile because her mother had cancer. Her fifth-grade home-room teacher pulled her out of class to encourage Emma to talk to her if she felt sad or worried. Other teachers tried to talk to Emma about her mother's situation and her feelings. Kids from school she didn't even really know stopped her in the hall to say, "My mom said I should check if you're OK." It may be really sweet, but Emma might have found it claustrophobic; there was no escape.

For the next decade, we assessed Emma as anxious, vigilant, listening for any comment that might signal a recurrence. At any mention of Liza's health, it seemed as if Emma's antennae shot up, wondering if this was the other shoe. On the other hand, Charlie seemed OK. He remained focused on school and what was coming up next in his life. "So you say Mom has cancer, but it's likely going to be OK? OK, thanks. Can I go play Xbox?"

Maybe our belief in our ability to communicate with children was overly confident. John was a professional at this. We always worked hard at communicating with our children. But as we discussed the breast cancer years later on with the kids, it became clear that they didn't understand as much as we thought they did. When a local magazine ran a piece on us in the spring of 2013, the writer emphasized that Liza's cancer was high risk, that in many ways she was lucky to be alive.[1] Both Charlie and Emma read the article, and for the first time they told us, a bit upset, that they had no idea Liza's cancer was that bad. Why didn't we tell them the truth?

We were taken aback at their reactions. How could they not have known? On further reflection, we realized that as they grew, and Liza did not die, we never formally revisited Liza's cancer with them. While the two of us rejoiced in landmark moments, two years, three years, five years, a big fiftieth birthday party, the kids did their kid things. No formal debrief, no repeat of the living room meeting. It turns out, we learned, that debriefs matter. Reopening the discussion at different stages of a child's maturation might be a good idea.

One more potential effect on our kids was Liza having genetic testing. Why had she, at the age of forty-three, gotten breast cancer and triple-negative at that? Because triple-negative is the type of cancer that appears in people with the BRCA gene, both Dr. Willey and Dr. Liu had recommended that she get tested. We knew that if

1 Rice, Alison, "The Big C," *Arlington Magazine*, vol. 3, no. 2, March–April 2013, pp. 74–81.

the testing found that Liza had a cancer-linked gene, then there was a 50 percent chance that each of the kids had it as well. That meant their risk for cancer was much higher than normal, and they could pass it on to their own children. We would have to figure out how and when to tell our children of their increased risk. The idea of telling our daughter that she was at risk for ovarian and breast cancer at an early age was daunting. Some girls who were informed of this went on to have hysterectomies and preventative mastectomies. No children of your own, no breasts. Or constant worry about *getting* cancer. Charlie was only slightly less of a concern. He'd have to tell any woman that he wanted to have children with of the risk of his passing the gene on to them. Was it fair to find out the information? Was it fair *not* to find out the information?

We were lucky. When the results came back a few weeks later, they reported that Liza did not have the BRCA1 or BRCA2 mutation, but they did note that Liza "may have an inherited predisposition to breast/ovarian cancer." It acknowledged that either it was possible that "there is a mutation present in the BRCA1 or BRCA2 genes that could not be detected by current techniques, although this chance is small." Finally, it cautioned that Liza should "[b]ear in mind that it is also possible that you may have an alteration in another cancer susceptibility gene that is very rare and/or has not yet been identified." So there's no obvious genetic cause for Liza's cancer, but not complete assurance that Charlie and Emma would not be predisposed to getting or passing on a gene for cancer. However, who really knows who is going to get cancer, and who isn't? It's a fear everyone lives with.

Maybe our kids were actually lucky that cancer has played such a large role in their lives. They already knew that life was unpredictable, and you just have to get on with it.

Epilogue

John and Liza here again.

Writing this book has forced us to reflect on our lives before, during, and after cancer. It has been a meaningful, mostly fun, sometimes difficult, and at times painful process for both of us. One of the things we have learned during the last fifteen years is that while our story has its own unique spin, it is not unique in the broader sense. Of course, intellectually we knew that—John's whole profession and much of Liza's volunteer life has been devoted to helping people with a similar story—but as the book relates, it's all personal now.

We are both glad that Liza didn't die, that our friends and families didn't have to endure the process of watching her decline and fade away, that she had the opportunity to see her children grow up. We have seen and experienced that particular trajectory too many times—sometimes from the periphery, sometimes close up. As we are writing this Epilogue, a twenty-three-year-old friend of Emma's is entering hospice for her final days, writing on her CaringBridge site about her experience of waiting for death from melanoma. We know that we have dodged a bullet—make that an IED—in our family, but we feel her family's pain more acutely because we have traveled down some of that road ourselves.

John became an oncologist in response to what he heard as God's call. He was pleased with having chosen a career that enabled him both to support his family and to serve others. It was only after Liza's cancer, after our journey through the dark valley, that he could see more clearly what his patients were going through. It was only then that he understood the real value of our healthcare system as well as the true personal impact he and his team were having on hundreds of patients each week. While he worked to provide every cancer patient the same care that Liza and he received, he came to realize that it was only a dream. Logistically, financially, interpersonally, it could never become reality. You can never really know what the experience is like until you've lived it yourself. Even with a vivid imagination, empathy has its limits. John found that after Liza's cancer, he could be a more effective guide for his patients and his team, but he failed to foresee the emotional fatigue that eventually would exhaust him when the objectivity and emotional distance that was essential to the doctor-patient relationship loosened up.

As for Liza, one of the long-term effects of having cancer is that, corny as it may seem, she has become more tolerant and more appreciative of the small things in life. Sure, she still swears at people on the road, on television, and on the Internet, but with every complaint, rant, or even fury, there is always a recognition: "I am lucky to be a part of this." Some things are harder to see that way than others, but the voice is always there: "Being here for this means being here for that." When someone on his or her birthday rues the fact that he or she is another year older, Liza frequently recites the familiar: "It beats the alternative."

So where did we end up as a couple in all of this? Our relationship has never been the type to engage in high drama, nor was it there during Liza's cancer treatment or during this book's writing. But symbolically, perhaps, we have handled both in the same way: We acted in parallel. Throughout the writing, a friend who read the drafts would ask each of us what we remembered about what the other one did during one event or another, how our relationship was affected, and remarking that we each seemed to leave the other out of our own narrative. Liza remembers that John was not terribly helpful in figuring out how to proceed, that he seemed to be hanging back. John remembers trying not to exert too much influence on decisions that were, in the end, going to have the greatest direct effect on Liza. In retrospect, it may appear as if this was a period of alienation, that maybe we didn't even like or trust each other during a time of great stress. But, in fact, we've always had deep respect and love for each other, and that frequently has manifested in each of us having the freedom to act without having to consult the other, a strong trust built over almost forty years of our lives together. After all that time, we frequently know what the other is thinking or feeling.

It is true that at the time of Liza's diagnosis, as we have recounted, we were more distant from each other, running on parallel tracks that were farther apart than they had been earlier. That's a common symptom of most romantic partnerships that have lasted more than twenty years and focused on caring for children, a dog, two para-keets, and aging parents. Liza's cancer brought us closer to each other and reminded us that having a partner to go through life with, even during the boring just-keep-the-kids-safe-get-the-laundry-done-food-on-the-table-and-moving-in-the-right-direction period, was for us the highest goal. We have been grateful that we have been able to do that since 2006. Our time together writing this book has re-confirmed our commitment to each other, to those suffering from cancer, and to God.

So why did Liza survive when many others don't? Not "why did God pick her?" We don't see God as a micro-manager, nor do we believe that God picks who lives and who dies based on some unknown points system or whim. But scientifically, why did Liza end up in the 50 to 60 percent of women diagnosed with triple-negative breast cancer whose cancer did not recur? Did she do more treatment than she really needed? Was she actually cured by the original surgery? Did the Adriamycin and Cytoxan do the job? Did they do it after four rounds instead of six? Was the platinum drug a miracle drug? Did the Zometa prevent breast cancer cells from invading her bones? Did the thirty-five rounds of radiation remove every last trace of cancer? Was the lack of a recurrence due to the increased exercise and the running? Perhaps it was the mediport, George Clooney, the beads, and the black cat. Maybe our faith made the difference.

Liza is reminded of her cancer and the treatment every day. She notices her appearance, particularly when her chest is uncovered. The scar on the right breast has tightened up over time, leaving a strange dent at the right underarm. She has neuropathy in the ends of her fingers, a side effect of the Taxol and platinum drugs. These nerve endings have been killed off, meaning that increasingly frequently, she can't feel things with them, particularly when it's cold. She finds it harder and harder to do certain actions, such as button a shirt, put on a necklace or earrings, or pick up small items. She drops things more and more often. As expected, her heart has sustained some damage from the Adriamycin. She entered menopause early, but because she had breast cancer, she is precluded from using hormone therapy to counter the effects of early menopause, such as vaginal dryness and premature loss of bone density. Eventually, she will have to have additional surgery on her breasts to replace the implants, which are made to last only about ten to fifteen years.

In the fifteen years since Liza's cancer, the field of cancer treatment has made great progress. New immune therapies, new drugs that target specific cancer pathways, and new diagnostic tools have improved survivals and lessened side effects. That decision she had to make about chemotherapy before or after surgery? It's no longer much of a decision. Almost all breast cancer patients receive chemotherapy first now. So many people are surviving their cancers that there is a new branch of oncology focused purely on survivorship, helping to restore cancer patients back to the "old" normal, or at least as close as possible. Liza's cancer dramatically reshaped John's practice of medicine. He no longer embraced the "more is better" approach that he had learned in training. It is no longer *how much* chemo patients can receive; it is now *how little* a patient can receive and get at least the same outcomes. Quality of life matters not only for those who are going to live, but also for those who are going to die.

For all of John's speeches and editorials, cancer care is not only still expensive, but also even more expensive. It's a luxury item, available only to those who can pay. On the positive side of the cost-benefit analysis, clinical research has become more efficient, more focused, and more designed to find larger improvements over less consequential small steps. Although cancer research funding is more evenly distributed across the tumor types, breast cancer is still the queen.

We will, however, be grateful forever to the breast cancer industrial complex, and we are sure it is their successes that allowed Liza to be alive today. Her fiftieth birthday party was a glorious celebration of her innovative treatments, her care team, and our realization that she was not going to die from breast cancer. To every patient nervously waiting on the next CT scan, we recommend throwing a small party if all is well at three years and a really big one at five years. In fact, to everyone who has overcome obstacles in life, from raising children to keeping a marriage together to caring for loved ones, remember that life itself is worth celebrating. Don't forget to celebrate, and in between the celebrations, don't forget to live.

As we finish this Epilogue, we are in quarantine, the death toll from COVID-19 is skyrocketing, and questions about when life will ever return to normal remain unanswered. Maybe in some way, everyone is experiencing a little of what cancer patients go through: the anxiety, the waiting game, the unrelenting uncertainty as to whether you will survive or not. Like cancer's unpredictability, we are unsure why some are getting infected, and some are not; why some are surviving seemingly unscathed, while others are dying in ICUs around the globe. But as cancer did for our relationship, we are hopeful that the pandemic will bring humanity closer together, remind us to value the simple joys of a hug, of sitting next to a friend over coffee, of family reunions, of sharing a bag of peanuts at a baseball game. We never know what lies ahead, so don't take anything for granted.

Acknowledgements

As this book attests, very few journeys through life are taken alone, or even with just two side by side. We are blessed with an incredible village of friends and family, too many to list by name, but each always there to support us, both then and now. However, there are a few who are directly responsible for this book.

We must first thank Alison Rice for writing such a lovely story about us for *Arlington Magazine* and Greg Hamilton for publishing it. It was this story that inspired our dear friend and accomplished writer and editor, Marianne Szegedy-Maszak, to suggest that we consider writing this book. And while the book took us many years to find the time to complete, Marianne was always its guardian angel, midwife, and editor, pushing us to make it better while simultaneously encouraging us to find our voices and holding our hands all along the way from the beginnings of the idea to its publication. This book would literally not exist without her.

We were finally able to find the time to write thanks to Georgetown University and its sabbatical program, which gave us a blessed four months in a quiet flat in Oxford, England atop Campion Hall, the Permanent Private Hall run by the Society of Jesus. Thank you to Reverend Dr. Nicholas Austin, the Master of Campion Hall, and to all those in the Campion Hall community for making us so welcome, to Trudi Preston for answering every question we had and solving every problem along with Alec Thorp, Sarah Gray, Mark Goodlake, and the Oxford IT crew, without all of whom we could not have functioned.

An enormous thank you to those who are mentioned in the book who cared for us both and to many who are not mentioned in the book but who cared for us both as well. A special thank you to Dr. Claudine Isaacs for being a consultant on all matters breast cancer both during and after Liza's treatment and during the writing of this book, and for being such a stalwart friend to both of us along with her entire family.

Thank you to Phil, Emmett and Annie Richardson for allowing us to share Holly's story. Thank you to all the patients and their caregivers who have taught us so many lessons and especially to those whose bravery and joy in the heat of battle remind us how we should be living every day.

Thank you to Barry Glassman, who seems to know absolutely the right person for everything, and who connected us with Rohit Bhargava of Ideapress. Rohit and his team masterfully and warmly guided us from a too long manuscript to publication, and we very much appreciate his taking this project on and shepherding it to market it so skillfully.

We could, of course, not have done any of this if not for our families, our parents, David, Jane, and Ginger Marshall and Charles and Betty Alexander, who brought us through difficult times in our lives with love and faith, and our siblings who supported us along the way: Lucy Alexander Murphy and her husband Braden who took over the day-to-day care of Liza's parents so that we could spend four months in England to work on this book; Elizabeth Marshall Taylor, David Marshall, Richard Edwins, and Elizabeth Edwins.

And most importantly, thank you to our children, Charlie and Emma Marshall. We feel so fortunate, that after a lifetime of unsolicited advice, cancer conversations, and forced marches through historic sites, that you still put up with us!